ICOG Campus

Imaging in Obstetrics and Gynecology

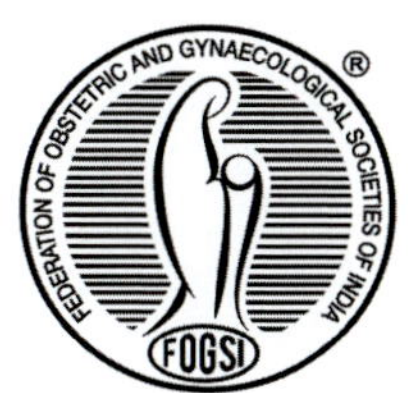

Indian College of
Obstetricians & Gynaecologists

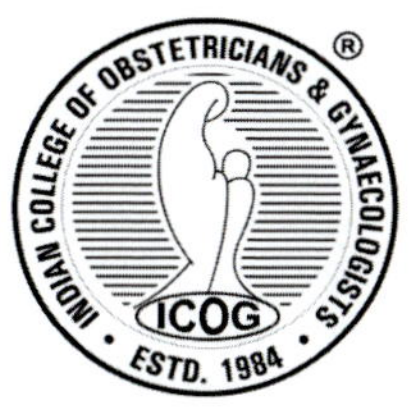

ICOG Campus

Imaging in Obstetrics and Gynecology

Sunita Tandulwadkar
President, FOGSI ICOG

Parag Biniwale
Chairperson, ICOG
Editor-in-Chief

Sarita Bhalerao
Secretary, ICOG

Ashok Kumar
Vice Chairperson, ICOG
Editor

Neha Pruthi Tandon
Co-Editor

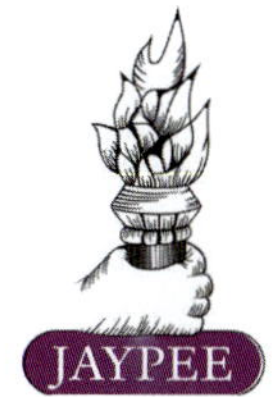

JAYPEE BROTHERS MEDICAL PUBLISHERS
The Health Sciences Publisher
New Delhi | London

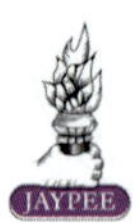 **Jaypee Brothers Medical Publishers (P) Ltd**

Headquarters
EMCA House, 23/23-B
Ansari Road, Daryaganj
New Delhi 110 002, India
Landline: +91-11-23272143, +91-11-23272703
+91-11-23282021, +91-11-23245672
e-mail: jaypee@jaypeebrothers.com

Corporate Office
4838/24, Ansari Road, Daryaganj
New Delhi 110 002, India
Phone: +91-11-43574357
Fax: +91-11-43574314
e-mail: jaypee@jaypeebrothers.com

Overseas Office
JP Medical Ltd
83 Victoria Street, London
SW1H 0HW (UK)
Phone: +44-20 3170 8910
e-mail: info@jpmedpub.com

EU GPSR Authorised Representative
Logos Europe, 9 rue Nicolas Poussin
17000, La Rochelle, France
Phone: +33 (0) 6 67 93 73 78
e-mail: contact@logoseurope.eu

Website: www.jaypeebrothers.com
Website: www.jaypeedigital.com

ICOG Campus—Imaging in Obstetrics and Gynecology

First Edition: **2026**

ISBN: 978-93-7202-075-5

Printed in India at Sterling Graphics Pvt. Ltd.

Contributors

Anshu Baser MS DNB FMAS (MUHS) MRCOG (London)
Consultant
Department of Obstetrics and Gynecology
Akash Hospital
Indore, Madhya Pradesh, India

Anusha MSR MBBS MS (OBG)
Consultant
Department of Fetal Medicine
Umarji Mother and Child Care Baner
Pune, Maharashtra, India

Archana Baser MS DNB FRCOG (London)
Consultant
Department of Obstetrics and Gynecology
Akash Hospital
Indore, Madhya Pradesh, India

Chinmay Umarji
MBBS DGO FRCOG MRCPI
Director
Umarji Mother and Child Care Baner
Pune, Maharashtra, India

Chinmayee Ratha MS FRCOG (UK) FIMSA FICOG Diploma in Fetal Medicine (FMF, UK)
Director and Lead Consultant
Department of Fetal Medicine
Fetal Resolution Clinic
Hyderabad, Telangana, India

Deepti Gupta MBBS MS DNB FICOG FMAS
Associate Professor
Department of Obstetrics and Gynecology
Netaji Subhash Chandra Bose Medical College, Jabalpur
Consultant and Unit Head
Ankur Fertility Clinic
Jabalpur, Madhya Pradesh, India

K Aparna Sharma MD DNB FICOG MNAMS
Professor
Department of Obstetrics and Gynecology
All India Institute of Medical Sciences
New Delhi, India

Pooja Holani Maheshwari
MBBS DNB
Clinical Fellow
Department of Fetal Medicine and Perinatology
Amrita Institute of Medical Sciences and Research Centre
Faridabad, Haryana, India

Pratik Tambe
MD FICOG FICRM FICMCH FIAOG
Governing Council Member
ICOG (2020–25)
Governing Council Member
ICRM (2024–26)
Chairperson, FOGSI Endocrinology Committee (2017–19)
Chairperson, AMOGS Endocrinology Committee (2020–24)
Managing Council Member
MOGS, ISAR, MSR

Priya Deshpande MBBS MS (OBGYN)
Fellowship in Fetal Medicine
Senior Consultant
Apollo Hospital, Navi Mumbai
Director
JIVVAM Fetal Medicine Center
Navi Mumbai, Maharashtra, India

Reema Bhatt MBBS MS DNB FICOG MNAMS Masters in Advanced Maternal Fetal Medicine
Professor and Head
Department of Fetal Medicine and Perinatology
Amrita Institute of Medical Sciences and Research Centre
Faridabad, Haryana, India

Rupal Parekh MBBS DNB (OBGY) DGO (Gold Medalist) Fetal Medicine Fellowship (ICOG)
Fetal Medicine Consultant
KIMS Hospital, Thane
Ex-Clinical Associate
Department of Fetal Medicine
Surya Mother and Child Hospital
Mumbai, Maharashtra, India

Tanisha Gupta MD
Senior Resident
Department of Obstetrics and Gynecology
All India Institute of Medical Sciences
New Delhi, India

Uday Thanawala
MD DGO FCPS DNB FICOG
Consultant
Department of Obstetrics and Gynecology
Thanawala Maternity Home and IVF Centre
Navi Mumbai, Maharashtra, India

Vandana Bansal MD DGO DNB MNAMS FICOG (Obstetrics and Gynecology) FRCOG (UK) FNB (High Risk Pregnancy and Perinatology)
Additional Professor
Nowrosjee Wadia Maternity Hospital
Seth GS Medical College, Mumbai
Director
Fetal Medicine Centre
Surya Mother and Child Hospital
Mumbai, Maharashtra, India

Message from Chairperson, ICOG

Imaging is a fundamental and constantly evolving tool in obstetrics and gynecology, providing crucial information for diagnosis, monitoring, and treatment. While ultrasound is the primary modality due to its safety, availability, and cost-effectiveness, magnetic resonance imaging (MRI) and computed tomography (CT) are also used for more complex cases and cancer staging.

Obstetric ultrasound has become a backbone of obstetric practice which helps clinical management better. The first-trimester 11-14-week scan would help assessing the baby for possible genetic abnormalities apart from prediction of preeclampsia, growth restriction, or preterm birth. The anomaly scan gives a survey of all organs giving information about structural malformation. The growth scans have shown important guidance for management of conditions like restricted fetus, or macrosomia.

Doppler ultrasound is a specialized application that measures and visualizes blood flow through vessels in the fetus, umbilical cord, and placenta. It is particularly valuable for monitoring high-risk pregnancies by assessing fetal well-being, screwing for preeclampsia, and detecting fetal hypoxia and anemia. This vital information aids clinical management and helps us plan suitable interventions at the right time.

In gynecology, ultrasound is the standard first-line imaging tool for evaluating the female pelvis. It can be performed transabdominally or transvaginally for higher resolution. It gives a great insight while assessing women for pelvic pain, evaluating women for heavy menstrual bleeding, assessing fertility, and differentiating complex masses. MRI is used to provide more detailed information than ultrasound, especially for evaluating the extent of gynecological cancers, diagnosing remote endometriosis, evaluating congenital uterine anomalies, and helping differentiate benign and malignant lesions.

I am sure this ICOG campus will give a correct insight into the emerging role of various imaging modalities. The contributors have given latest recommendations based on current literature and I am sure the readers will be immensely benefitted with help in decision-making whenever there is a dilemma. I appreciate efforts taken by Dr Ashok Kumar, Vice Chairperson, ICOG, and Dr Neha Pruthi Tandon as editors of this book.

Parag Biniwale
Chairperson, ICOG
Editor-in-Chief

Preface

Imaging has revolutionized the practice of obstetrics and gynecology, transforming diagnosis, management, and outcomes for women's health worldwide. With rapid advances in ultrasound, Doppler, CT, MRI, and PET, clinicians are now equipped with sharper tools than ever before to guide evidence-based care.

Campus on Imaging in Obstetrics and Gynecology brings together comprehensive knowledge and practical insights to provide a complete reference for medical students, postgraduate trainees, radiologists, and practicing obstetricians and gynecologists. Organized systematically, it covers—core principles of imaging and their application to female reproductive health, obstetric imaging, including early pregnancy evaluation, fetal growth, placental disorders, and intrapartum assessments.

It provides a guidance on which gynecologic imaging is better in malignant pathologies of the uterus, cervix, and ovary.

With contributions from experts in the field, this text supports better diagnostics, safer interventions, and improved maternal and reproductive outcomes.

Whether for a student preparing for examinations, a postgraduate refining diagnostic acumen, or a clinician seeking practical imaging pearls, this book offers a definitive guide to contemporary imaging in women's health.

Ashok Kumar
Neha Pruthi Tandon

Acknowledgments

We would like to express our heartfelt gratitude for this book to our guide, *Dr Parag Biniwale*, Chairperson, ICOG, for his unwavering support, invaluable insights, and constant encouragement throughout the compilation of the book. We are also thankful to *Dr Sarita Bhalerao*, Secretary, ICOG, for her cooperation and support in publishing this book.

We would also like to thank our visionary President, *Dr Sunita Tandulwadkar*, President, FOGSI ICOG, who has given a freehand and encouraged each and every FOGSIan to come forward and do wonders for the health of women. Our sincere thanks go to Dr Suvarna Khadilkar, Secretary General, FOGSI for always supporting and giving strength to us.

We wish to express our sincere appreciation to each contributor whose profound insights and tireless dedication have significantly enriched the content of this book.

A special note of thanks goes to our esteemed institution Atal Bihari Vajpayee Institute of Medical Sciences and Dr Ram Manohar Lohia Hospital, New Delhi, India, whose cooperation and encouragement have been instrumental in the realization of this project.

We express our sincere appreciation to the team at M/s Jaypee Brothers Medical Publishers (P) Ltd, New Delhi, India for their outstanding support and professionalism. In particular, we thank Mr Ankit Vij (Managing Director), Mr Sabyasachi Hazra (Director, PG and PNR Content), and Mr Akhilesh Saxena (Development Editor) for their tremendous efforts in bringing this book to fruition.

Ashok Kumar
Neha Pruthi Tandon

Acknowledgments

Contents

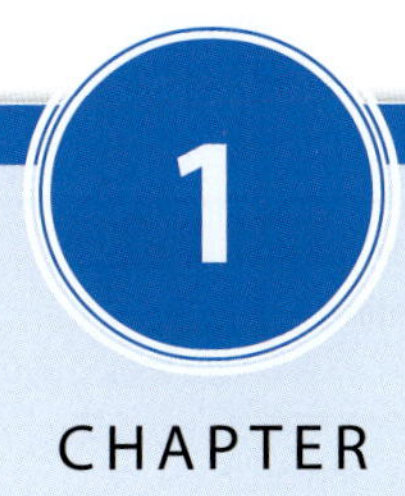

CHAPTER

Basic Principles of Imaging Modalities

Chinmay Umarji, Anusha MSR

INTRODUCTION

Imaging is so much incorporated in the routine obstetrics and gynecology (OBG) that it is difficult to think of OBG in the absence of the same. Imaging modalities in OBG include X-ray with or without fluoroscopy, mammography, ultrasound with B-modes, M-mode and Doppler studies, computed tomography (CT) with or without contrast, magnetic resonance imaging (MRI) with or without contrast, and positron emission tomography (PET) scan. We have tried to simplify the basic principles of imaging modalities in this chapter.

X-RAYS, MAMMOGRAPHY, AND FLUOROSCOPY

Principle

They are electromagnetic waves that are produced when the cathode is in the form of a filament which emits electrons on heating. The anode is made of solid copper molybdenum and is called the target. The filament is made up of tungsten and coiled to provide high resistance to the current. The electrons produced are changed into X-rays on hitting the anode and getting stopped. Cooling oil is led in and out of the hollow of the anode to maintain low temperature **(Fig. 1)**. The lead shield absorbs stray X-rays.[1]

Contrast Agents

Iodine-based and barium-sulfate compounds are used in X-ray and CT imaging exams.

Fluoroscopy

Fluoroscopy is a study of moving body structures-similar to an X-ray "movie". A continuous X-ray beam is passed through the body part being examined. The beam is transmitted to a TV-like monitor so that the body part and its motion can be seen in detail.

CLINICAL APPLICATIONS IN OBSTETRICS AND GYNECOLOGY

- Hysterosalpingography for tubal testing also provides some information about the shape of the uterus rules out mullerian abnormalities.

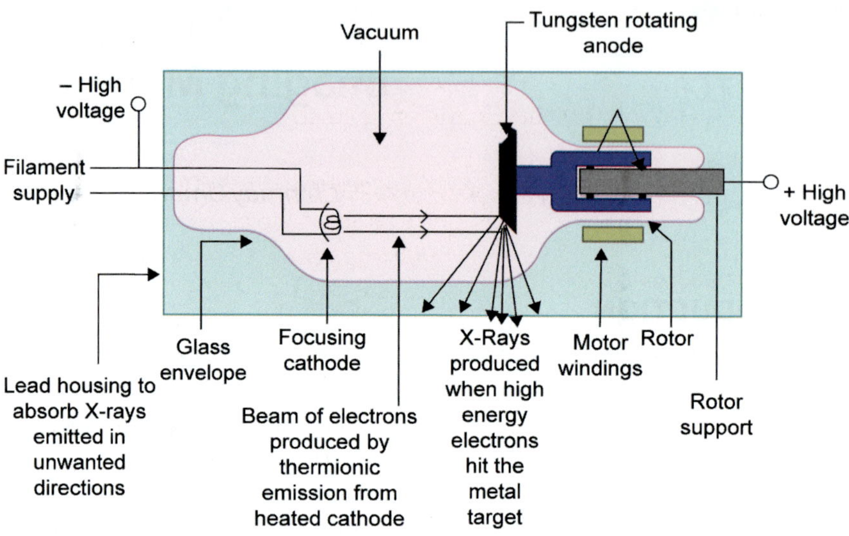

Fig. 1: How X-ray is generated.

- Uterine and internal lilac embolization in obstetrics for postpartum hemorrhage (PPH) can be used for T4 (Tone, tissue trauma and thrombin) e.g., traumatic PPH as in cases of supralevator broad ligament hematoma, PAS (Placenta accreta spectrum), atonic uterus and DIC. In gynecology, used in treatment of fibroid, adenomyosis, therapeutic to control excessive bleeding in cancer cervix patients and control postoperative bleeding.
- Fallopian tube catheterization under fluoroscopy guidance - useful technique for proximal tubal blockage.
- Mammography, for routine screening of breast and classify lesions as per BIRADS scoring.
- Abdominal erect X-ray and chest X-ray for diagnosis of bowel problems especially after surgery where peritoneal cavity was opened, any chronic cough or serious respiratory illness.
- X-ray can be done safely with abdominal shielding if clinically indicated as the dose of radiation exposure is less than 0.1 m curie.
- *Advantage:* Quick, convenient, potable non-invasive, painless and relatively inexpensive
- *Disadvantage:* Ionizing radiation, poor soft tissue detail and 2D imaging.

ULTRASOUND SOUND

This modality of imaging uses sound waves; the waves are transmitted through medium by local displacement of particles within medium by compression & rarefaction. Speed of sound depends on the medium in which they are travelling and temperature – Air 343 m/s, Water 1482 m/s, Steel 5960 m/s.

Average in biological tissue 1540 m/s.[2] Hence the need for application of gel on the probe so the air pockets are avoided. Sound is measured by frequency hertz (Hz) = cycles/sec. Human audible range of sound includes 20 Hz to 20,000 Hz (20 kHz), ultrasound frequencies above audible range that is 20,000 Hz.

USG machine consists of different probes connected to the machine. Inside the probe there are piezoelectric crystals which are made up of quartz, zirconium titanate, and modern ceramics. When an electric current is applied to a crystal, they change shape rapidly and produce waves which are ultrasound. The probe sends these ultrasound waves into the patient body at each boundary of different tissues; some of the waves are reflected back to the probe which records the position and strength of these echoes. The scanning unit combines this information to create an image of the boundaries of tissues and organs in which the sound waves are reflected from the ultrasound machine calculates the depth of each wave by measuring the time taken by each sound wave to return **(Fig. 2)**. Fluids don't reflect the sound waves; this

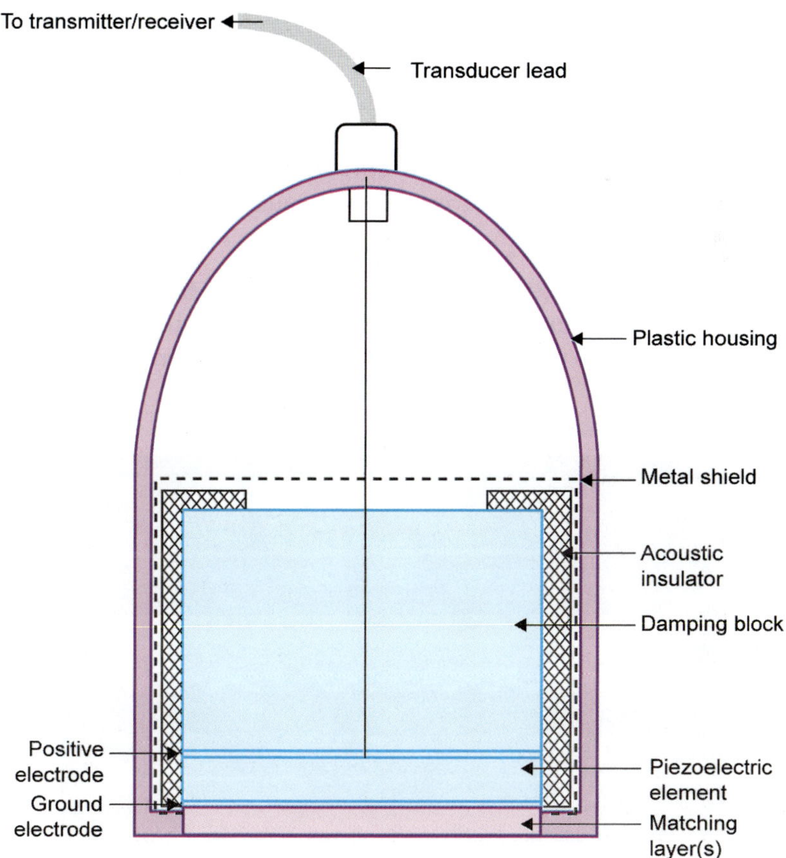

Fig. 2: Ultrasound probes.

principle is used in obstetric USG where amniotic fluid acts as the acoustic window and the fetal parts are better seen.[3]

USG probes come in different sizes and shapes and have different clinical implications, hence USG is sonographer dependent. Probes and the connection to the machine are the most fragile, expensive and delicate in the machine, hence require special care during handling.

Distance of reflector is calculated (time window send-receive) D = ½ Time of flight x velocity.

Probes producing precise images have higher frequency and are limited by depth of the penetration, whereas the probes with lower frequency produce lesser resolution with deeper penetration of the image.

For example, 3.5 MHz will travel 10–20 cm, 5.0 MHZ = 5–10 cm, 7.5 MHz = 2–5 cm

10.0 MHz = 1–4 cm respectively

Footprint of the image depends on the probe selected; linear probe gives rectangular, curvilinear probe gives c shaped footprint and transvaginal probe gives small c shaped. Attenuation as the sound waves travel through tissue, their energy decreases due to absorption, reflection and refraction. When there is a large area, a greater number of sectors, more depth, angle and width ultrasound waves take time.

Echogenicity: Different tissues reflect sound waves differently,

- *Hyperechoic:* Brighter, due to more amount of sound waves reflected
- *Hypoechoic:* Due to some waves reflected, muscle
- *Anechoic:* Will appear dark no waves reflected as in fluids filled structure.

M-Mode (Motion): The variations in a single line of echoes are recorded against time. These are used in the measurement of fetal heartbeat and study the conducting system of the fetal heart to detect fetal arrhythmia **(Fig. 3)**.

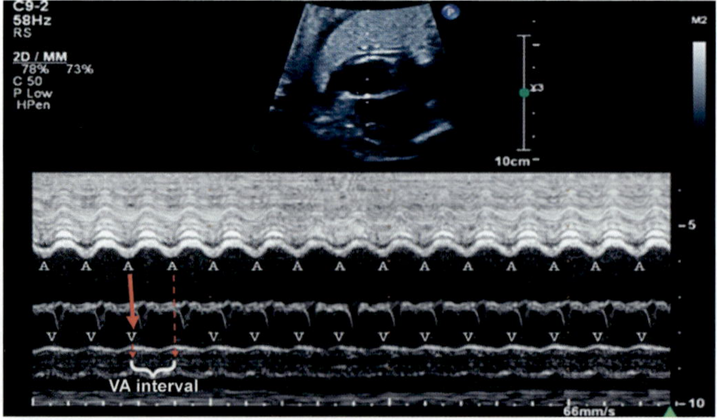

Fig. 3: M-mode of USG.

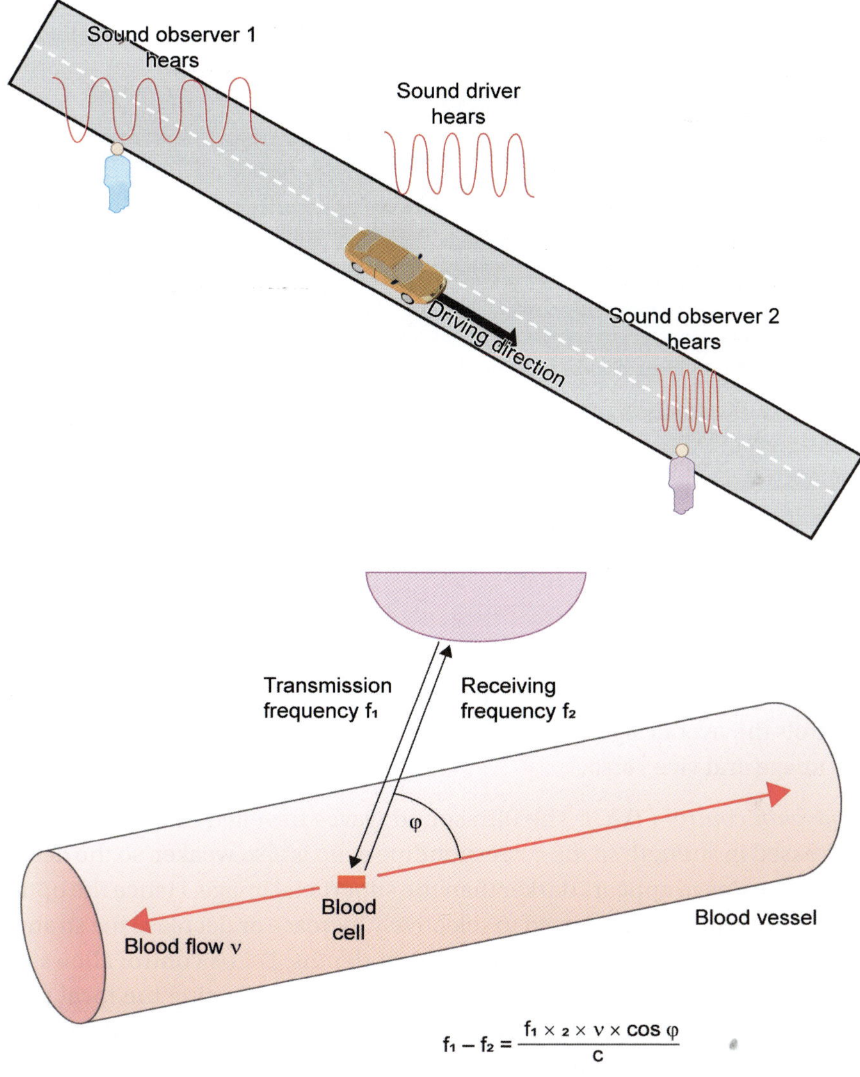

Fig. 4: Doppler principle.

Doppler USG: It relies on the phenomenon of Doppler effect, which states the difference in the frequency of the waves changes whether something is moving towards the probe and away from the probe. The USG machine measures the shift in the frequency and is used to measure the blood flow, mostly represented as color. In addition to color Doppler we also have pulsed wave Doppler and power Doppler.[4] Doppler studies are controlled by the gate width, Pulse repetition frequency, baseline, angle correction, sweep speed and high pass filter **(Figs. 4 and 5)**.

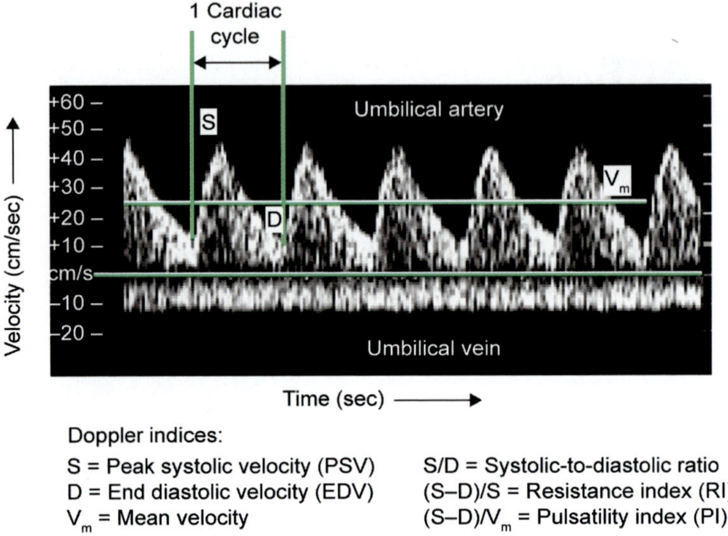

Fig. 5: Doppler indices.

Knobology: Understanding the controls for better image generation is essential. Power output controls the strength of the signal of the probe; gain controls the overall signal amplified example the higher the gain the brighter the image and vice versa.

Time gain control (TGC): The ultrasound waves travelled into the depth are decreased in strength so the corresponding echo is also weaker, so the deeper part of the image appears darker than the superficial image. Hence the option of TGC control should be used to selectively increase or decrease the strength of the different amount of gain at different depths. Focus control allows you to get the detailed image of the area of interest by adjusting the focal point of the beam. Depth control defines the depth of the visible area of the interest to be studied **(Fig. 6)**. The field of view controls the resolution of the image; a narrower field has better resolution that is used to study the fetal heart.[5]

Image artefacts: An ultrasound image which does not match actual anatomy, there are many artefacts like

- *Drop out/acoustic shadowing:* Dark area posterior to dense reflector, mostly marked along US beam. Hence the area behind the fetal bones and behind the calcified fibroids appear as drop outs. This can be reduced or removed by adjusting angle of insonation.
- *Posterior enhancement/amplification:* Area of increased brightness immediately posterior to cystic structure, this is caused by lack in sound attenuation through a structure with few interfaces.

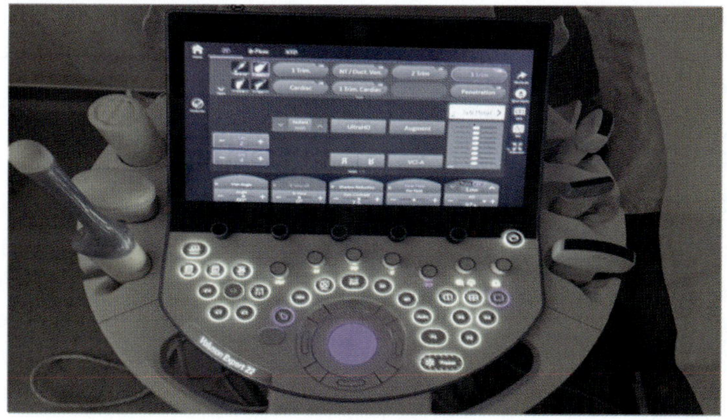

Fig. 6: Knobology.

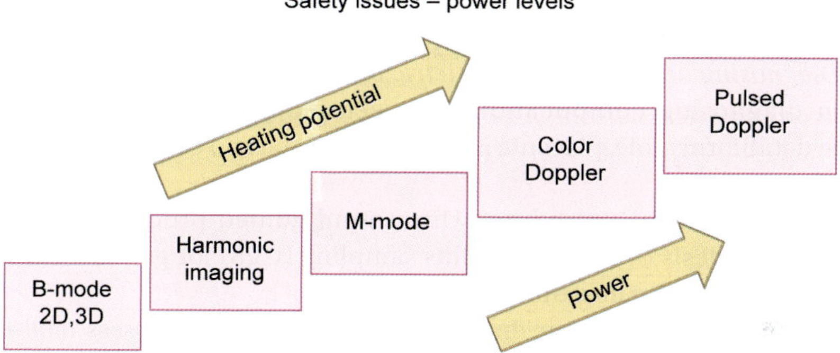

Fig. 7: Safety issues.

- *Reverberation:* It occurs when a US beam encounters 2 strong parallel reflectors, multiple parallel echoes result from back-and-forth travel of US between 2 reflecting surfaces. It is reduced by changing the angle of insonation.
- *Side lobe artifact:* Results from strong reflector that lies outside the incident beam, but within the side lobe of the central beam, resulting in incorrect information.

Safety issues: Although USG is safer it can cause certain issues if not done correctly. Increase in movement of molecules can result in rise in temperature. The USG machine calculates this as Thermal Index = TI (<1.0) (power needed to increase temperature by 1°C), it should be kept as low as possible. Doppler especially pulse wave increases the TI significantly hence should be avoided in the first trimester **(Fig. 7)**.

Mechanical Index = MI (<1.0)

ALARA principle—as low as reasonably achievable, means the strength of the signal should be as low as possible and for the shortest duration as possible.[6]

Clinical Application of USG in OBG

In Obstetrics

- *First trimester:* Confirming pregnancy, viability, location, estimating the gestational age, detecting multiple Pregnancies, early fetal anomaly survey NT scan and screening for preeclampsia with Doppler studies.
- *Second trimester:* Fetal anatomy scan, along with information about placental location, screening for preterm delivery by transvaginal cervical length assessment.
- *Third trimester:* Assessing fetal growth and wellbeing, detecting fetal position, doppler studies for assessment of fetal growth problems, fetal position in the uterus, liquor assessment and delayed anomaly assessment.
- *Diagnosing and managing obstetric complications:* Ultrasound is used in diagnosing complications like ectopic pregnancy, miscarriage, hydatidiform mole, placenta previa, vasa previa, and complication of twin pregnancy.
- *guiding invasive procedures:* Ultrasound guided procedures such as amniocentesis or chorionic villus sampling (CVS) for genetic testing or fetal therapy, like intrauterine transfusions
- *Monitoring during labor:* Intrapartum ultrasound can assess fetal head station and position, aiding in the management of labor and potentially increase the safety of the instrument application for assisted vaginal delivery.

In Gynecology

Evaluating the uterus, ovaries, and fallopian tubes: Ultrasound helps diagnose and manage conditions like uterine fibroids, ovarian cysts, and endometriosis.

- *Assessment of pelvic organs:* Uterus MUSA, Endometrium by IETA and ovary by IOTA scoring systems.
- *Assessing pelvic pain:* It aids in diagnosing the cause of pelvic pain, including ectopic pregnancy, pelvic inflammatory disease, and ovarian torsion.
- *Fertility assessments:* Ultrasound is used to monitor follicular development and guide egg retrieval during assisted reproductive technologies.
- *Detecting and characterizing pelvic masses:* Ultrasound can detect and classify adnexal masses, including distinguishing between cysts and solid tumors, which is crucial for conditions like ovarian cancer and pelvic floor dysfunction.

Advanced Ultrasound Technologies

Recent advancements in ultrasound technology, such as high-resolution ultrasonography, Doppler ultrasound, 3D/4D ultrasound, and the integration of artificial intelligence (AI), are further enhancing its capabilities in both obstetrics and gynecology.

Safety and Limitations

Limitations: It's important to remember that ultrasound cannot identify all fetal abnormalities, and the quality and accuracy of the images can be affected by factors like operator skill, patient body habitus, and the presence of amniotic fluid. Ultrasound should always be performed when medically indicated and in conjunction with clinical judgment. Hence Usg should be used when indicated and follow the ALARA principles.

Magnetic Resonance Imaging

Magnetic resonance imaging (MRI) is very safe, has no radiation and gives better resolution. It uses a static magnetic field the strength of which is measured by Tesla, its available as 1.5 tesla and 3 tesla's. The more the tesla the better the resolution and also shorter application time. It uses the principle that your body is made up of water and has H_2O, two protons of hydrogen when subjected to strong magnetic fields and then a short radiofrequency pulse is sent. This is detected by a receiver coil(s) placed around the region of interest, and Fourier transformation produces an image. Image contrast can be weighted to analyze specific structures **(Fig. 8)**. Each tissue returns to its

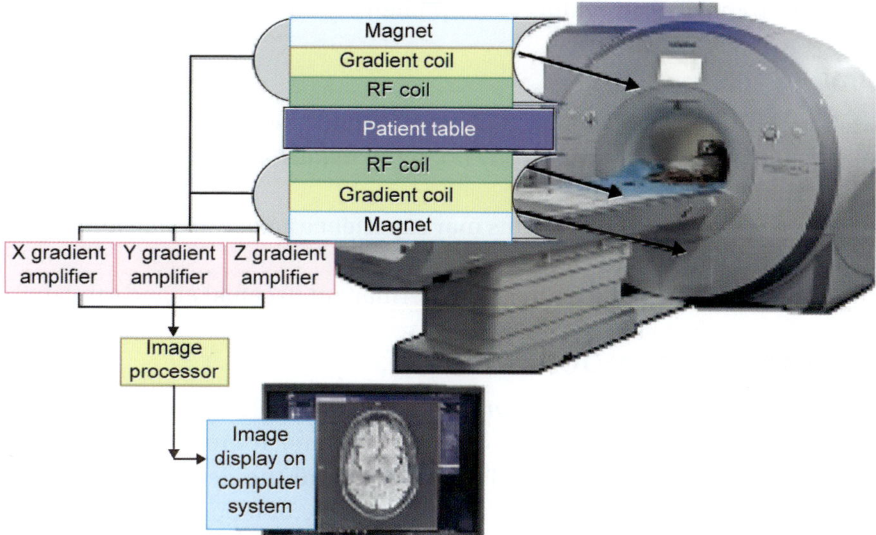

Fig. 8: Principles of magnetic resonance imaging.[8]

resting state via a combination of T1 and T2 relaxation: T1 is the time required to regain longitudinal magnetization and T2 is the transverse relaxation time.[7]

Clinical Applications in Obstetrics

- *Fetal anomalies:* Fetal MRI especially in the second trimester is very safe. It provides additional information in Fetal CNS abnormalities, fetal CDH, in management of single fetal demise of MCMD twins, and especially when ultrasound findings are inconclusive which are affected by oligohydramnios and maternal BMI.
- MRI helps diagnose and evaluate placenta accreta spectrum
- *Maternal Complications:* Conditions like appendicitis, pelvic masses, and other issues during pregnancy, especially when ultrasound is limited.

Clinical Applications in Gynecology

- *Uterine abnormalities:* For mapping of fibroids, endometriosis prior to planning any intervention.
- *Ovarian cysts:* MRI helps in differentiate the indeterminate mass on IOTA scoring on USG and guide treatment decisions.
- *Congenital anomalies:* MRI is the imaging modality of choice for evaluating congenital malformations of the female reproductive tract.

KEY ADVANTAGES OF MRI

- *Non-ionizing radiation:* Making it safe for use during pregnancy.
- Excellent Soft Tissue Detail.
- *Multiplanar imaging:* MRI can produce images in multiple planes (axial, sagittal, coronal), providing a comprehensive view of the pelvic organs.

Limitations

- *Cost:* MRI is generally more expensive than ultrasound.
- *Availability:* MRI scanners may not be as readily available as ultrasound machines.
- *Claustrophobia:* Some patients may experience anxiety or claustrophobia in the MRI machine.
- Cannot be used in the patient with permanent pacemaker and implants.

COMPUTER TOMOGRAPHY

There are two processes of absorption: The photoelectric effect and the Compton effect. The particular case of computer tomography (CT), the emitter of X-rays rotates around the patient and the detector, placed on diametrically opposite sides, picks up the image of a body section (beam and detector move in synchrony). Unlike X-ray radiography, the detectors

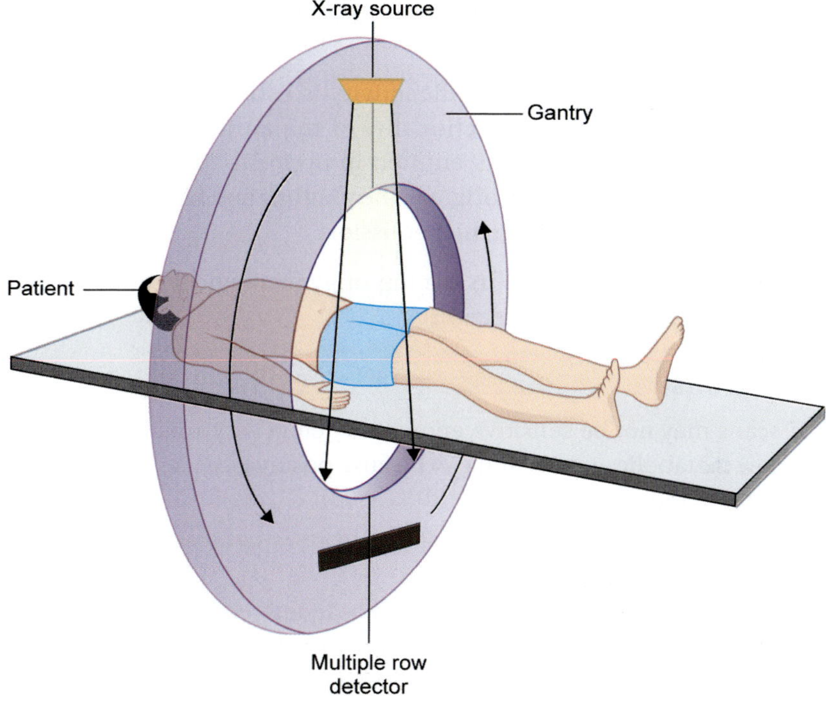

Fig. 9: Principles of CT scan.

of the CT scanner do not produce an image. They measure the transmission of a thin beam (1–10 mm) of X-rays through a full CT of the body **(Fig. 9)**. The image of that section is taken from different angles, and this allows us to retrieve the information on the depth (in the third dimension).[9]

Clinical application in OBG is mostly limited to gynecology where it is used for staging malignancy of the female reproductive system, guiding biopsy procedures and its use in obstetrics is limited due to radiation exposure. In obstetrics when suspicion of pulmonary venous thrombosis exists CT angiography should be planned with abdominal shield. CT brain can be considered to rule out CNS pathologies.

PET SCAN

The principle of positron emission tomography (PET) is that radiation emitted from a radiopharmaceutical injected intravenously into a patient is registered by external detectors positioned at different orientations. The isotope distributes within different tissues according to the carrier molecule (isotopic labeling) and emits a positron (a positively charged electron).

This positron in turn interacts with a free electron and an annihilation reaction occurs, resulting in the production of two 511-KeV photons emitted at almost 180° to each other.

Then, the distribution of radioactivity is estimated by (filtered) back projection methods. The directionality of the annihilation photons (two 511-keV annihilation photons emitted in opposite directions) provides a mechanism for localizing the origin of the photons and hence, the radioactive decay process that resulted in their emission.[10]

Clinical application in obg: In staging of gynecological cancer, treatment response and recurrence detection

Limitations

PET scans may not be sensitive enough to detect very small lesions or those with low metabolic activity and can be false positive due to infection. There is a risk of radiation exposure.

CONCLUSION

Imaging is the backbone of medicine, it has redefined the way we understand the anatomy, physiology and pathology of any disease. Imaging without radiation hazards like Ultrasound and MRI can be safely used in pregnancy. Fetal imaging has helped us ensure the health and well-being of the developing fetus, provide early diagnosis and management of fetal abnormalities and optimize pregnancy outcomes for both mother and baby. In gynecology it helps to make diagnosis, plan management options, plan surgery better and optimize the well being of women.

KEY POINTS

- *X-rays and fluoroscopy:* Quick, inexpensive, useful in HSG, embolization for PPH, tubal interventions, mammography; limited by radiation and poor soft-tissue detail.
- *Ultrasound (USG):* Backbone of OBG imaging; safe, real-time, versatile (B-mode, M-mode, Doppler); central for pregnancy scans, fetal growth, anomalies, and gynecological evaluation.
- *Knobology and safety:* Proper use of controls, recognition of artefacts, and adherence to ALARA principle (TI <1, MI <1) ensure safe, accurate imaging.
- *MRI:* Radiation-free, high-resolution, multiplanar imaging; valuable for fetal CNS, PAS, gynecological masses, and congenital anomalies; limited by cost, access, and implants.
- *CT and PET:* Reserved mainly for gynecological oncology staging, treatment response, and recurrence detection; use in obstetrics is restricted due to radiation exposure.

- *Misconception and counseling:* Many patients still fear or opt for termination after X-ray/CT exposure in pregnancy. It is crucial to counsel that diagnostic doses are usually well below harmful thresholds, and unnecessary termination should be avoided.

REFERENCES

1. Seeram E. (2023). Basic Radiation Physics for Diagnostic X-Ray Imaging. In: X-Ray Imaging Systems for Biomedical Engineering Technology. Springer, Cham. https://doi.org/10.1007/978-3-031-46266-5-2
2. http://www.isuog.org/StandardsAndGuidelines/Statements+and+Guidelines/Safety+ statements
3. https://www.isuog.org/education/basic-training.html
4. Bhide A, Acharya G, Bilardo CM, Brezinka C, Cafici D, Hernandez-Andrade E, Kalache K, Kingdom J, Kiserud T, Lee W, Lees C, Leung KY, Malinger G, Mari G, Prefumo F, Sepulveda W and Trudinger B. ISUOG Practice Guidelines: use of Doppler ultrasonography in obstetrics. Ultrasound Obstet Gynecol. 2013;41: 233-9.
5. https://www.isuog.org/education/basic-training.html, lecture 2 on Transducers, Image Production, Knobology and Scanning Planes.
6. Ultrasound in pregnancy. Practice Bulletin No. 175. American College of Obstetricians and Gynecologists. Obstet Gynecol. 2016;128: e241–56. Obstetrics & Gynecology 128(6):p e241-e256,2016. | DOI: 10.1097/AOG.0000000000001815
7. Story L, Rutherford M. Advances and applications in fetal magnetic resonance imaging. The Obstetrician & Gynaecologist. 2015;17:189-99.
8. Joao Tourais, Chiara Coletti, Sebastian Weingärtner, Chapter 1 - Brief Introduction to MRI Physics, Editor(s): Mehmet Akçakaya, Mariya Doneva, Claudia Prieto, Advances in Magnetic Resonance Technology and Applications, Academic Press, Volume 7, 2022, Pages 3-36, ISSN 2666-9099, ISBN 9780128227268, https://doi.org/10.1016/B978-0-12-822726-8.00010-5.
9. Pelberg, Robert. (2015). Basic Principles in Computed Tomography (CT). 10.1007/978-1-4471-6690-0_2.
10. Pawar AA, Patil DB, Patel S, Mankad M, Dave P. Role of PET-CT Scan in Gynaeconcology. J Obstet Gynaecol India. 2016;66(5):339-44. doi: 10.1007/s13224-015-0681-1. Epub 2015 May 5. PMID: 27486279; PMCID: PMC4958067.

CHAPTER

Imaging in Pregnancy

Reema Bhatt, Pooja Holani Maheshwari

INTRODUCTION

Imaging in pregnancy presents a clinical conundrum—while essential for diagnosis and monitoring, it must be performed with utmost caution to avoid fetal harm. Over recent decades, technological advancements, evolving guidelines, and medicolegal awareness have amplified the role of imaging in obstetric care **(Table 1)**. While non-ionizing modalities such as ultrasound and MRI are widely accepted as safe, the judicious use of ionizing imaging remains crucial to avoid potential teratogenic or carcinogenic effects[7,12]

TABLE 1: Imaging modalities in pregnancy.[4,7]

Modality	*Radiation Type*	*Safety in Pregnancy*	*Common Indications*
Ultrasound (USG)	Non-ionizing	Safe	Viability, dating, anomalies, Doppler studies
Transvaginal USG	Non-ionizing	Safe	Early pregnancy, cervical length
MRI	Non-ionizing	Safe (avoid gadolinium)	CNS anomalies, placental invasion
X-ray	Ionizing	Use with shielding	Chest conditions
CT Scan	Ionizing	Use with caution	Trauma, appendicitis
Nuclear medicine	Ionizing	Rarely used	Pulmonary embolism (V/Q scan)
Fluoroscopy	Ionizing	Use sparingly	GI procedures, rare interventions

1. American College of Obstetricians and Gynecologists. Guidelines for Diagnostic Imaging During Pregnancy and Lactation. Obstet Gynecol. 2017;130(4):e210–e16.
2. Brent RL. Saving lives and changing family histories: appropriate counseling of pregnant women and men and women of reproductive age, concerning the risk of diagnostic radiation exposures during and before pregnancy. Am J Obstet Gynecol. 2009;200(1):4-24

NON-IONIZING MODALITIES

Ultrasonography (USG)

Ultrasonography is a cornerstone in obstetric imaging due to its safety, accessibility, and diagnostic value. As a non-ionizing modality, it poses no known teratogenic risk when used judiciously. All ultrasound examinations during pregnancy should adhere to the ALARA (As Low As Reasonably Achievable) principle to limit acoustic exposure and thermal effects. Appropriate below configuration of ultrasound machines and proper clinical indications ensure fetal safety.[1]

- *FDA intensity limit:* 720 mW/cm^2[1,7]
- *Thermal effects:* Theoretical temperature rises up to 2°C, primarily with Doppler modes.
- *Safety profile:*
  - *B-mode:* Safest with minimal thermal risk.
  - *Color/Spectral Doppler:* Higher thermal potential but safe when clinically justified **(Table 2)**.

Ultrasound imaging, when clinically indicated and appropriately configured, does not pose a measurable risk to fetal development.[2] It remains the first-line modality for assessment throughout gestation, especially in high-risk pregnancies.

Magnetic Resonance Imaging (MRI)

MRI is a non-ionizing imaging modality that offers excellent soft tissue contrast and is not operator-dependent. It is preferred over CT in pregnancy for soft tissue evaluation due to the absence of radiation. MRI is considered safe during all trimesters of pregnancy[3] **(Table 3)**.

Human Study Finding[5]

- No significant increase in birth defects or cancer with first-trimester MRI.
- Slight increase in rheumatologic/skin conditions with gadolinium exposure.
- Stillbirth/neonatal death is higher in the gadolinium group (adjusted RR 3.70).
- Gadolinium use during pregnancy should be limited to cases where benefits clearly outweigh risks.

Clinical Applications of MRI in Pregnancy

- Appendicitis (preferred over US if available)
- Placental abnormalities
- Fetal anomalies when US is inconclusive
- Maternal pelvic pathology

TABLE 2: Clinical applications of ultrasonography in pregnancy.[1,7]

Gestational age/ indication	*Ultrasound application*	*Purpose*
Early pregnancy (≤10 weeks)	Transvaginal USG: Crown–Rump Length (CRL)	• Confirm intrauterine pregnancy • Accurate dating • Detect fetal cardiac activity
Ectopic pregnancy	Transvaginal USG	Identify extrauterine gestation (tubal, cervical, ovarian, abdominal)
First trimester screening (11–13+6 weeks)	• NT measurement • Nasal bone assessment • Ductus venosus and tricuspid flow • Combined with serum markers (PAPP-A, β-hCG)	Aneuploidy risk estimation (e.g., Trisomy 21)
Mid-trimester anomaly scan (18–22 weeks)	Detailed fetal anatomy scan • Placental evaluation	• Detect structural anomalies (NTDs, cardiac, renal) • Placental location and morphology
Growth monitoring (≥28 weeks)	• Biometric parameters (BPD, HC, AC, FL) • Amniotic fluid (AFI/SDP) • Fetal Doppler studies (Umbilical, MCA, uterine arteries)	• Assess fetal growth trends • Detect IUGR, macrosomia, fluid abnormalities
High-risk pregnancies	• Transvaginal USG for cervical length • Serial growth/Doppler scans	Monitor conditions like preeclampsia, GDM, IUGR, and multiple gestations
Procedural Guidance	Real-time USG	Safe execution of CVS, amniocentesis, and cordocentesis

1. Salomon LJ, Alfirevic Z, Da Silva Costa F, et al. ISUOG Practice Guidelines: Ultrasound assessment of fetal biometry and growth. Ultrasound Obstet Gynecol. 2019;53(6):715-23.
2. Brent RL. Saving lives and changing family histories: appropriate counseling of pregnant women and men and women of reproductive age, concerning the risk of diagnostic radiation exposures during and before pregnancy. Am J Obstet Gynecol. 2009;200(1):4-24.

IONIZING MODALITIES

X-ray Imaging During Pregnancy

X-ray is a ionizing imaging modality. Diagnostic X-ray procedures are occasionally warranted during pregnancy for urgent maternal indications

TABLE 3: MRI safety in pregnancy.[7]	
Concern	*Summary*
Radiation	MRI uses magnetic fields, not ionizing radiation
Teratogenesis	No human evidence; animal data mostly negative
Tissue heating	Minimal near uterus; negligible concern
Acoustic damage	No fetal harm reported
Trimester consideration	No special restriction for first trimester

Brent RL. Saving lives and changing family histories: appropriate counseling of pregnant women and men and women of reproductive age, concerning the risk of diagnostic radiation exposures during and before pregnancy **(Table 4)**. Am J Obstet Gynecol. 2009;200(1):4-24.

TABLE 4: Use of MRI contrast agents.	
Type	*Safety Considerations*
Gadolinium-based	Crosses placenta; teratogenic at high/repeated doses in animals; minimal human data; use only if essential
Superparamagnetic iron oxide	No data on fetal safety; not recommended during pregnancy

Brent RL. Saving lives and changing family histories: appropriate counseling of pregnant women and men and women of reproductive age, concerning the risk of diagnostic radiation exposures during and before pregnancy. Am J Obstet Gynecol. 2009;200(1):4-24.

such as trauma or suspected serious pathology. The fetal radiation dose from most single diagnostic X-ray procedures is substantially lower than the threshold for deterministic effects.[4]

- X-rays may be used during pregnancy when medically necessary, or may occur before pregnancy is diagnosed.
- The fetus receives about 1 mGy of background radiation throughout pregnancy.
- Radiation risk depends on gestational age at exposure and radiation dose.
- Exposure >1 Gy during early embryogenesis (first 2 weeks) can be lethal.
- High-dose exposure can cause growth restriction, microcephaly, and intellectual disability.
- The central nervous system is most vulnerable between 8–15 weeks of gestation.
- Intellectual disability has a threshold of 60–310 mGy; lowest dose reported causing it is 610 mGy.[4,7]

- Diagnostic X-rays rarely reach these dose levels.
- No reported increase in anomalies, growth restriction, or miscarriage below 50 mGy.
- For exposures >50 mGy, counseling and targeted prenatal imaging are advised.
- Carcinogenesis risk is very low; 10–20 mGy may increase leukemia risk 1.5–2 times over baseline.
- Termination should not be recommended solely based on diagnostic radiation exposure.
- For multiple imaging studies, consult a radiation physicist to estimate fetal dose.
- Breastfeeding is not affected by external diagnostic X-rays and can continue safely.

Computed Tomography

CT is a form of ionizing radiation and generally delivers higher fetal doses than conventional radiography, diagnostic scans typically result in fetal exposures well below the threshold.[7,12]

- CT should not be withheld if clinically indicated; benefits and risks must be discussed.
- In emergencies (e.g., appendicitis, bowel obstruction), maternal benefit often outweighs fetal risk.
- MRI should be considered if equally effective and timely available, due to its safety.
- Radiation dose from CT varies with protocol and image spacing.
- CT pelvimetry can expose the fetus to up to 50 mGy, but low-dose protocols reduce it to ~2.5 mGy.
- CT of the chest (e.g., for suspected pulmonary embolism) results in lower fetal radiation than V/Q scan.
- Spiral CT delivers radiation doses similar to conventional CT when used typically.

Contrast Media in CT

- Oral contrast agents are not absorbed systemically and are safe in pregnancy.
- Intravenous iodinated contrast helps visualize vessels and soft tissue.
- *Common side effects:* Nausea, vomiting, flushing, injection site pain; rare—anaphylactoid reactions.
- Iodinated contrast can cross the placenta but has shown no teratogenic/mutagenic effects in animal studies.

- Concerns about fetal thyroid effects from iodide exposure are not supported by human studies.
- Contrast should only be used when essential for diagnosis that impacts care.

Nuclear Medicine Imaging

Nuclear medicine imaging in pregnancy involves the administration of radiopharmaceuticals tagged with gamma-emitting radioisotopes to assess physiological function. Among these, *technetium-99m* is the most frequently employed isotope due to its favorable physical properties, including a *short half-life of 6 hours* and emission of *only gamma radiation*, which minimizes fetal exposure.[6]

- It evaluates physiological organ function using radio labeled compounds.
- Hybrid imaging systems combine nuclear imaging with CT to enhance diagnostic accuracy.
- Fetal exposure depends on properties of the radioisotope used.
- Technetium-99m is the most commonly used isotope in pregnancy (e.g., V/Q scan, renal, bone scans).
- Typical fetal dose from technetium-99m procedures is <5 mGy, considered safe.
- Technetium-99m has a 6-hour half-life and emits only gamma rays, minimizing radiation dose.
- Radioactive iodine (iodine-131) is contraindicated during pregnancy due to fetal thyroid toxicity, especially after 10–12 weeks of gestation.
- Technetium-99m should be used instead of iodine-131 if thyroid imaging is necessary.
- Radionuclides are excreted in breast milk in variable amounts **(Table 5)**.

RADIATION SAFETY AND GUIDELINES

Recommendations:

- *ACOG & ACR:* Diagnostic X-rays are not contraindicated if clinically warranted.
- Termination is not advised for exposures below 5 rad.
- Use shielding and optimized settings to reduce fetal dose.

Radiation protection:

- Lead shielding (abdomen, thyroid)
- Lowest effective dose
- Prefer non-ionizing methods when possible **(Tables 6 and 7)**.

TABLE 5: Fetal radiation dose[7,11]

Type of examination	***Fetal dose* (mGy)***
Very low-dose examinations (<0.1 mGy)	
Cervical spine radiography (AP and lateral views)	< 0.001
Head or neck CT	0.001–0.01
Radiography of any extremity	< 0.001
Mammography (two views)	0.001– 0.01
Chest radiography (two views)	0.0005–0.01
Low- to moderate-dose examinations (0.1–10 mGy)	
Radiography	
Abdominal radiography	0.1–3.0
Lumbar spine radiography	1.0–10
Intravenous pyelography	5–10
Double-contrast barium enema	1.0–20
Computed tomography (CT)	
Chest CT or CT pulmonary angiography	0.01–0.66
Limited CT pelvimetry (single axial section at femoral heads)	<1
Nuclear medicine	
Low-dose perfusion scintigraphy	0.1–0.5
Technetium-99m bone scintigraphy	4–5
Pulmonary digital subtraction angiography	0.5
Higher-dose examinations (10–50 mGy)	
Abdominal CT	1.3–35
Pelvic CT	10–50
^{18}F PET/CT whole-body scintigraphy	10–50

* Fetal exposes varies with gestational age, maternal body habitus and exact acquisition parameters.

Note: Annual average background radiation = 1.1-2.5 mGy. ^{18}F = 2-[fluorine-18] fluoro-2-deoxy-D-glucose. Modified from Tremblay E, Therasse E, Thomassin-Naggara I, Trop I. Quality initiatives: guidelines for use of medical imaging during pregnancy and lactation.

1. Brent RL. Saving lives and changing family histories: appropriate counseling of pregnant women and men and women of reproductive age, concerning the risk of diagnostic radiation exposures during and before pregnancy. Am J Obstet Gynecol. 2009;200(1):4-24.
2. McCollough CH, Schueler BA, Atwell TD, et al. Radiation exposure and pregnancy: when should we be concerned? Radiographics. 2007;27(4):909-17.

TABLE 6: Decision-making – termination after radiation exposure.

Guideline	*Recommendation*
Danish Rule (1959)[8]	Termination if fetal dose >10 rad
Wagner et al.[9]	Consider termination >5 rad (organogenesis); >15 rad likely
Hall et al. (1991)[10]	Consider termination >10 rad (10 days–26 weeks)

1. Andersen A. Radiation and pregnancy: a survey of the problem of irradiation in relation to pregnancy. Acta Radiol. 1959;51:89-98.
2. Wagner LK, Lester RG, Saldana LR. Exposure of the pregnant patient to diagnostic radiations: A guide to medical management. 2nd edition. Madison (WI): Medical Physics Publishing; 1997.
3. Hall EJ, Giaccia AJ. Radiobiology for the Radiologist. 4th edition. Philadelphia: J.B. Lippincott; 1991.

TABLE 7: Effects of gestational age and radiation dose on radiation induced teratogenesis [4,7,11]

Gestational period	*Effects*	*Estimated threshold dose**
Before implantation (0–2 weeks after fertilization)	Death of embryo or no consequence (all or none)	50–100 mGy
Organogenesis (2–8 weeks after fertilization)	• Congenital anomalies (skeleton, eyes, genitals) • Growth restriction	200 mGy 200–250 mGy
Fetal period	***Effects***	***Estimated Threshold dose****
8–15 weeks	• Severe intellectual disability (high risk)† • Intellectual deficit • Microcephaly	60–310 mGy 25 IQ-point loss per 1,000 mGy 200 mGy
16–25 weeks	Severe intellectual disability (low risk)	250–280 mGy

* Data based on animal studies, epidemiologic evidence from atomic bomb survivors, and medical radiation exposure cases (e.g., uterine cancer radiotherapy).

† High risk due to rapid neuronal development and migration in the 8–15 week window.

1. American College of Obstetricians and Gynecologists. Guidelines for Diagnostic Imaging During Pregnancy and Lactation. Obstet Gynecol. 2017;130(4):e210-e16.
2. Brent RL. Saving lives and changing family histories: appropriate counseling of pregnant women and men and women of reproductive age, concerning the risk of diagnostic radiation exposures during and before pregnancy. Am J Obstet Gynecol. 2009;200(1):4-24.
3. McCollough CH, Schueler BA, Atwell TD, et al. Radiation exposure and pregnancy: when should we be concerned? Radiographics. 2007;27(4):909-17.

KEY POINTS AND CONCLUSION

- Imaging during pregnancy plays a vital role in maternal-fetal care and should be performed with careful consideration of both maternal indications and fetal safety.
- Ultrasound and MRI, being non-ionizing, are the preferred imaging modalities throughout pregnancy and carry no proven risk when used appropriately.
- Ionizing imaging (X-ray, CT, nuclear medicine) can be used when clinically indicated, especially in maternal emergencies, with precautions to minimize fetal exposure.
- Fetal radiation risks are highly dependent on gestational age and dose received. Most diagnostic imaging procedures deliver radiation doses well below teratogenic thresholds.
- Imaging in the first trimester requires greater caution due to organogenesis and increased sensitivity of the CNS, particularly between 8–15 weeks.
- Gadolinium-based contrast agents and iodinated contrast media should be used only when essential, after weighing potential risks and benefits.
- Termination of pregnancy should not be recommended based solely on diagnostic radiation exposure; decisions must be individualized with support from a radiation physicist and maternal-fetal medicine specialist.
- Effective communication and counseling are crucial to help patients and clinicians understand the actual risks, which are often overestimated.
- Follow the ALARA principle and use shielding, low-dose protocols, and alternative modalities wherever feasible.

REFERENCES

1. Patel SJ, Reede DL, Katz DS, Subramaniam R, Amorosa JK. Imaging the pregnant patient for nonobstetric conditions: algorithms and radiation dose considerations. Radiographics. 2007;27:1705-22.
2. Ultrasonography in pregnancy. ACOG Practice Bulletin No. 101. American College of Obstetricians and Gynecologists. Obstet Gynecol. 2009;113:451-61.
3. Theilen LH, Mellnick VM, Longman RE, Tuuli MG, Odibo AO, Macones GA, et al. Utility of magnetic resonance imaging for suspected appendicitis in pregnant women. Am J Obstet Gynecol. 2015;212(3):345.e1-6.
4. American College of Radiology. ACR–SPR practice parameter for imaging pregnant or potentially pregnant adolescents and women with ionizing radiation. Resolution 39 . Reston (VA): ACR; 2014.
5. Leyendecker JR, Gorengaut V, Brown JJ. MR imaging of maternal diseases of the abdomen and pelvis during pregnancy and the immediate postpartum period. Radiographics. 2004;24:1301-16.
6. Adam A, Dixon AK, Gillard JH, Schaefer-Prokop CM, editors. Grainger & Allison's diagnostic radiology: a textbook of medical imaging. 6th edition. New York (NY): Churchill Livingstone/Elsevier; 2015.

7. The American College of Obstetricians and Gynecologists (ACOG) Committee Opinion No. 723, titled Guidelines for Diagnostic Imaging During Pregnancy and Lactation, offers evidence-based recommendations on the safe use of imaging modalities in pregnant and lactating patients was initially published in October 2017 and reaffirmed in 2021.
8. Hammer-Jacobsen E. Therapeutic abortion on account of X-ray examination during pregnancy. Danish Medical Bulletin. 1959;6(7):221-6.
9. Wagner LK, Lester RG, Saldana LR. "Exposure of the pregnant patient to diagnostic radiations: a guide to medical management." Medical Physics Publishing; 1997.
10. Hall EJ. Radiobiology for the Radiologist. 4th edition. Philadelphia: J.B. Lippincott; 1991.
11. Tremblay E, et al. Imaging Pregnant and Lactating Patients: Radiologists Role in Counseling and Decision Making 2012;32(3):897-911.
12. ICRP. Pregnancy and medical radiation. ICRP Publication 84. Ann ICRP. 2000:30.

CHAPTER

Ultrasonography at 11–14 Weeks of Gestation

K Aparna Sharma, Tanisha Gupta

INTRODUCTION

Ultrasound examination between 11 and 14 weeks of gestation is a vital part of modern obstetric practice. Originally performed mainly to confirm fetal viability and determine gestational age, the scan is now seen as a comprehensive evaluation that provides important information about fetal health and pregnancy risks. A routine check during this time helps confirm viability and multiple pregnancies, ensure accurate dating, screen for aneuploidy, detect major structural anomalies early, and assess the risk for preterm preeclampsia. The key advantage of the 11–14 weeks ultrasound is its dual purpose: it reassures the expectant mother while enabling early detection of high-risk conditions. This enables timely counseling, preventive measures, and personalized pregnancy care. This chapter outlines the objectives, technical details, and current guidelines for performing and documenting the 11–14 weeks ultrasound.

OBJECTIVES OF THE 11–14 WEEKS SCAN

The first-trimester scan performed at 11–14+0 weeks of gestation, corresponding to the crown rump length (CRL) of 45–84 mm, serves several purposes as listed in **Table 1**.

TABLE 1: Objectives of the 11–14 weeks scan.[2]

- *Confirmation of viability*—demonstration of cardiac activity, assessment of fetal heart rate
- *Accurate dating*—CRL measurement provides the most precise estimation of gestational age, with an error margin of ±5–7 days, superior to later biometric measurements[1]
- *Determination of chorionicity and amnioticity* in multiple pregnancies—crucial for prognosis and follow-up
- *Screening for aneuploidy*—via nuchal translucency and other sonographic markers, often combined with maternal serum biochemistry
- *Screening for preeclampsia*—using maternal characteristics, mean arterial pressure, biochemical markers, and uterine artery Dopplers
- *Early detection of major anomalies*—certain severe structural abnormalities can be diagnosed at this stage

PRE-EXAMINATION COUNSELING

All pregnant women should be offered an 11–14 weeks scan. Before starting the scan, the woman or couple should be counselled regarding the potential benefits and limitations of the first-trimester ultrasound. This discussion is an important part of good clinical practice and helps ensure informed participation in the examination

EQUIPMENT

The 11–14 weeks ultrasound requires high-quality equipment with advanced software, compounding technology, and high-resolution transducers. Both transabdominal (2–9 MHz) and transvaginal (9–12 MHz) probes should be available, with the choice depending on image quality and maternal factors such as body mass index. The system must allow real-time 2D grayscale imaging, M-mode, color/power Doppler, and spectral Doppler, though Doppler use should be limited to clear clinical indications. Adjustable acoustic power controls are essential, and examinations should follow the as low as reasonably achievable (ALARA) principle with thermal and mechanical indices kept below 1.0.[3] The machine should also have freeze-frame and zoom functions, electronic calipers, and facilities for image storage, recording, and printing. Regular maintenance and servicing are necessary to ensure optimal performance and safety.

GUIDELINES FOR EXAMINATION

Assessment of Viability

In early pregnancy, viability is confirmed by the demonstration of fetal cardiac activity on ultrasound. Cardiac activity is usually seen from 5–6 weeks of gestation using 2D B-mode imaging. The fetal heart rate can be measured with M-mode or spectral Doppler and should be recorded after assessment over several cycles.[2] The rate normally rises until around 10 weeks (mean ~171 bpm) and then decreases slightly by 14 weeks (mean ~156 bpm).[4] Abnormally high or low heart rates may indicate aneuploidy or structural cardiac abnormalities, and should be reassessed during the examination

Biometry and Dating of the Pregnancy

Crown–rump length (CRL) **(Fig. 1)** should be measured as part of the routine first-trimester scan, either transabdominally or transvaginally. This is the most accurate method to establish or confirm gestational age up to 13 + 6 weeks, with an accuracy of ± 5–7 days, except in pregnancies conceived by in-vitro fertilization, where the conception date is already known.[1] The measurement should follow standard criteria: the fetus oriented horizontally, in a neutral position (neither flexed nor hyperextended), with the image magnified to fill

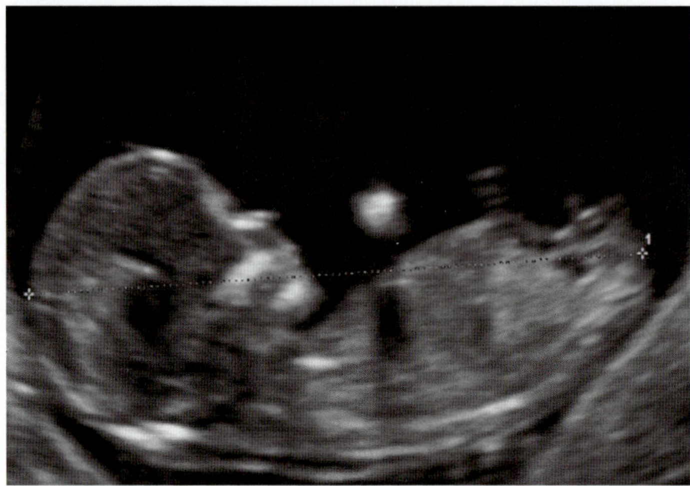

Fig. 1: Crown rump length (CRL) measurement at 11–14 weeks scan.

most of the screen.[2] Calipers are placed on the crown and rump endpoints, which must be clearly visualized. When multiple CRL measurements are obtained, gestational age should be based on the best-quality measurement between 45 and 84 mm.[2] It is important to note that reduced CRL may be seen in fetuses with trisomy 18 or triploidy. Dates should not be adjusted to 'normalize' growth in such cases, particularly if structural anomalies are also present. When the CRL is greater than this length (84 mm), other biometry indices can be used (head circumference, biparietal diameter, abdominal circumference, or femur length)

Screening for Aneuploidy

One of the primary objectives of performing an 11–14 weeks prenatal sonographic scan is to detect fetal structural anomalies and markers that can be used to assess the risk of chromosomal defects. Several sonographic markers can be used, and standardization of these measurements has been shown to increase their reliability and reproducibility. These markers are often combined with maternal serum biochemistry and maternal characteristics to refine risk assessment for aneuploidy. The commonly assessed markers are:

- Nuchal translucency (NT)
- Nasal bone (NB)
- Ductus venosus (DV) flow
- Tricuspid regurgitation (TR)

Raised nuchal translucency (NT) detects about 70% of trisomy 21 cases. The combined test, which incorporates maternal age, NT, and serum biochemistry (PAPP-A and β-hCG), performed between 11 and 13 + 6 weeks, significantly improves detection, with rates of approximately 82–87%.[5]

Nuchal Translucency

Nuchal translucency (NT) refers to the sonographic appearance of subcutaneous accumulation of fluid behind the fetal neck in the first trimester of pregnancy **(Fig. 2)**. The incidence of chromosomal and other abnormalities is related to the size of NT, rather than its mere presence. Reliable NT measurement depends on appropriate training and strict adherence to a standardized technique to ensure uniformity of results among different operators. The optimal gestational age for measurement is 11 + 0 to 13 + 6 weeks, when the fetal crown-rump length (CRL) measures 45–84 mm. The correct, standardized technique for NT measurement was first described by Nicolaides and colleagues, and forms the basis of international guidelines (FMF, ISUOG) and is described in **Table 2**.[2,6] Neck position significantly affects measurement: Hyperextension can increase NT by ~0.6 mm, and flexion can decrease NT by ~0.4 mm. An abnormal NT is defined as a measurement of ≥3.0 mm or greater than the 95th centile for the corresponding CRL.

Nasal Bone

The nasal bone is evaluated in the same midsagittal section as NT, using a magnified image that includes the echogenic tip of the nose and the rectangular palate anteriorly. Posteriorly, the translucent diencephalon and the nuchal membrane are also seen **(Fig. 2)**. The nasal bone lies just beneath the echogenic skin line of the face and should normally appear more echogenic than the overlying skin at the nasal tip and bridge. On a correct image, three distinct lines are visible:

1. The upper echogenic line represents the skin.

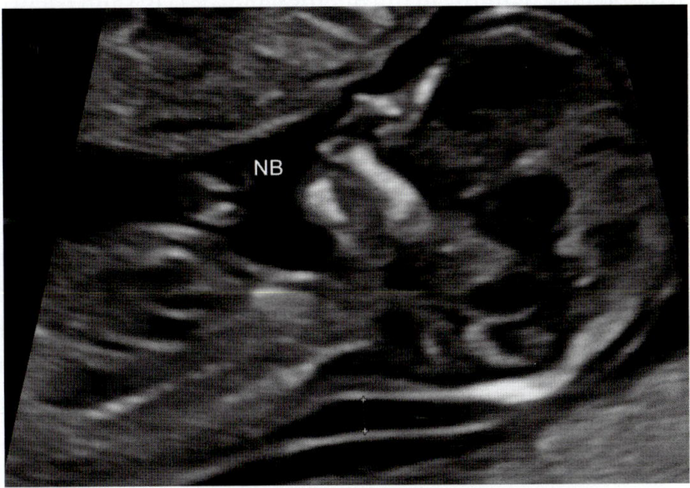

Fig. 2: Midsagittal view of fetal face, demonstrating nuchal translucency and nasal bone (NB) measurements.

TABLE 2: Requirements for nuchal translucency (NT) measurement at 11–14 weeks scan.[2,6]

- Gestation 11–13+6 weeks and crown–rump length 45–84 mm
- The midsagittal plane and fetus must be in a neutral position
- Magnified such that only the fetal head and upper thorax should be included, and calipers measure 0.1 mm increments
- The maximum thickness of subcutaneous translucency between the skin and soft tissue overlying the cervical spine should be measured
- Calipers should be placed on the lines that define NT thickness ("on-to-on measure")
- More than 1 measurement should be taken, and the maximum should be reported
- Demonstration of the fetus separate from the amnion to ensure the appropriate space is measured

2. The thicker, brighter lower line corresponds to the nasal bone.
3. A third line, in continuity with the skin but at a higher level, represents the nasal tip.

If the nasal bone is not more echogenic than the skin, it is considered hypoplastic or absent. Delayed ossification leading to hypoplasia or absence between 11 + 0 and 14 + 0 weeks is a strong sonographic marker for aneuploidy, particularly trisomy 21. The nasal bone is absent in 60–70% of fetuses with trisomy 21, about 50% in trisomy 18, and 30% in trisomy 13, but is rarely absent in euploid fetuses.[7] Therefore, its assessment provides high positive and negative likelihood ratios in first-trimester screening.

Ductus Venosus and Tricuspid Flow

Abnormal blood flow patterns in the ductus venosus (DV) and tricuspid valve are important markers at the 11–14 weeks scan. These reflect underlying structural or functional cardiac defects often associated with aneuploidy. In the DV, normal flow **(Fig. 3A)** shows forward velocity during systole (S-wave), diastole (D-wave), and atrial contraction (a-wave). An absent or reversed a-wave, or an increased pulsatility index for veins (PIV), is considered abnormal. Such changes are seen in about 80% of trisomy 21 fetuses but only in ~5% of euploid pregnancies.[8] Assessment is performed in a right paramedial sagittal section with color Doppler to identify the vessel, and a small pulsed-wave gate (≈1 mm) to record the waveform.[2] Tricuspid flow **(Fig. 3B)** is assessed in the four-chamber view using pulsed-wave Doppler across the tricuspid valve. Tricuspid regurgitation, defined as retrograde flow >60 cm/s for more than 50% of the cardiac cycle, is rare in euploid fetuses' but frequent in aneuploidy, particularly trisomy 21.[9] Both DV flow and tricuspid regurgitation are highly valuable when integrated with nuchal translucency and biochemical markers for first-trimester risk assessment.

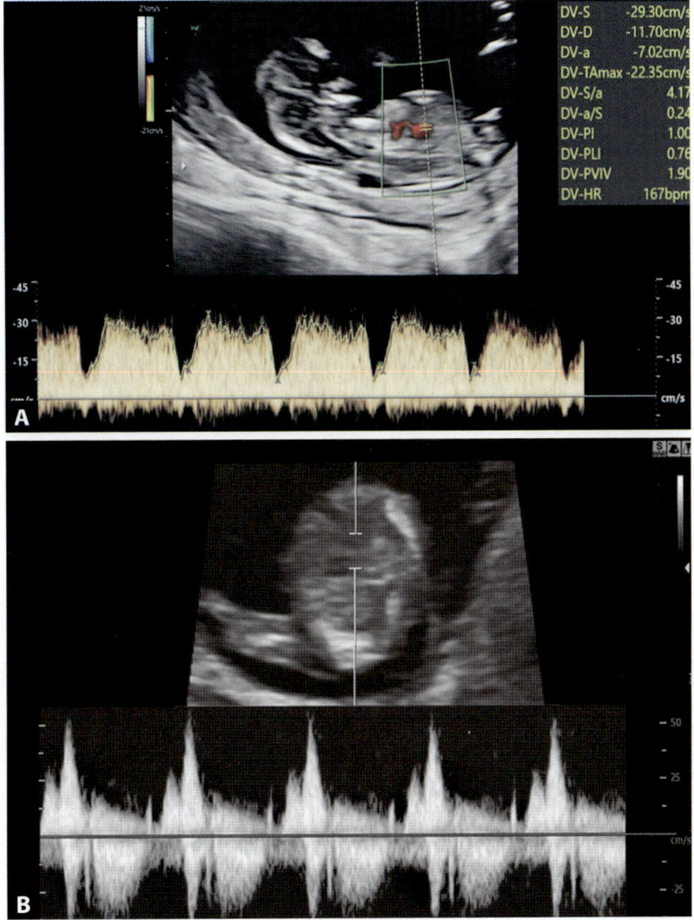

Figs. 3A and B: Ductus venosus and tricuspid valve waveform.

Screening for Preeclampsia

The optimal approach to first-trimester screening for preeclampsia is through the Fetal Medicine Foundation (FMF) algorithm, which combines maternal history, risk factors, mean arterial pressure (MAP), uterine artery pulsatility index (UtA-PI), and biochemical markers such as placental growth factor (PlGF) available at https://fetalmedicine.org/research/assess/preeclampsia. This integrated model provides the highest predictive accuracy for early-onset disease with a detection rate of 89.7%.[10] To obtain UtA-PI, a midsagittal view of the uterus is acquired to identify the cervical canal and internal os **(Fig. 4)**. With the probe kept in the midline, gentle tilting to each side helps localize both uterine arteries at the level of the internal os using color Doppler. A 2-mm pulsed-wave Doppler gate is then placed to encompass the entire vessel, ensuring an angle of insonation <30°. Once three uniform consecutive waveforms are recorded, the pulsatility index (PI)

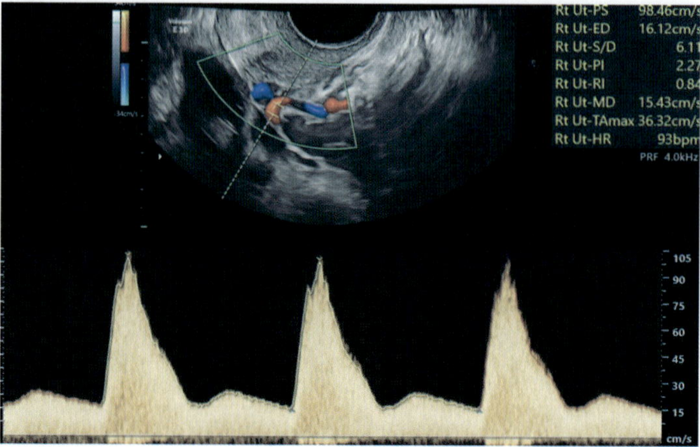

Fig. 4: Uterine artery Doppler velocity waveforms.

BOX 1: The 11–14 weeks scan.

- *Confirm:* Viability, plurality, and chorionicity
- *Date:* Use CRL for the most accurate gestational age
- *Screen:*
  - *Aneuploidy:* NT, nasal bone, ductus venosus, tricuspid flow + biochemistry
  - *Preeclampsia:* FMF algorithm (history, MAP, UtA-PI, PlGF)
- *Detect anomalies:* Apply basic or detailed ISUOG checklists; up to 40–66% of major anomalies detectable
- *Assess maternal structures:* Placenta, cervix, uterus, and adnexa
- *Key requirement:* High-resolution equipment, standardized protocols, and trained operators

is measured using automatic tracing.[2] The mean PI of both uterine arteries is then calculated and incorporated into the risk assessment algorithm.

Early Detection of Major Anomalies

A key role of the 11–14 week scan is the early detection of fontal structural anomalies **(Box 1)**. While not all abnormalities are visible this early, a significant proportion can be recognized, allowing timely counseling and management **(Figs. 5A to R)**. Studies suggest that 40–66% of major anomalies may be detected in the first trimester. ISUOG recommends two structured approaches for anomaly screening:

1. **Basic (Minimum) Checklist:** This approach ensures that all essential structures are assessed, providing reassurance in low-risk pregnancies and identifying major abnormalities. The basic checklist is described in **Table 3**.
2. **Detailed (Best Practice) Checklist (Table 4).**

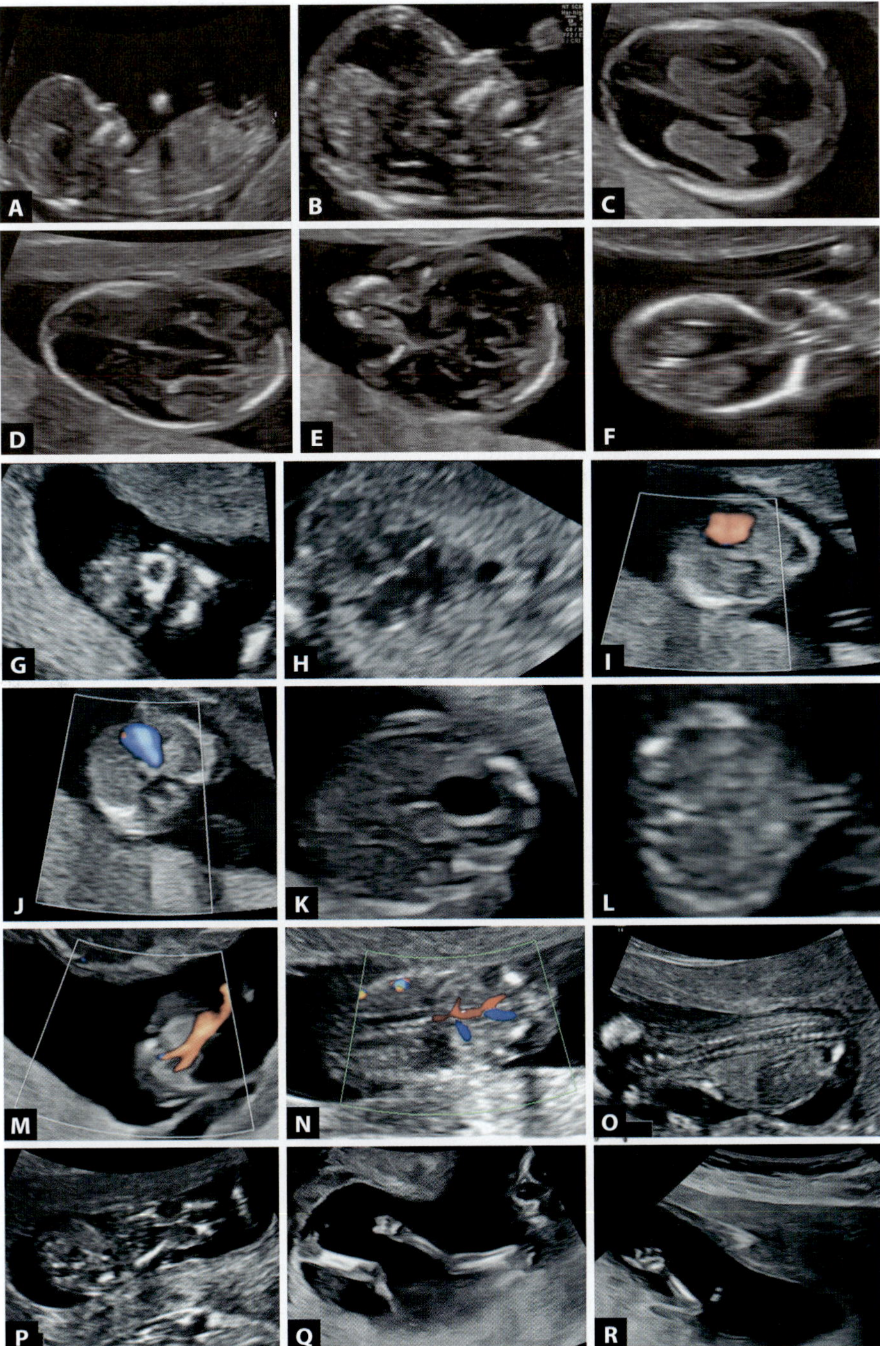

Figs. 5A to R: Fetal anatomy at first trimester scan. (A) CRL; (B) NT/NB; (C) IHF with choroid plexus cyst; (D) Transcerebellar view; (E) and (F) Transorbital view; (G) Retronasal triangle; (H to J) 4 C heart, inflows, outflow; (K) Stomach; (L) Cord insertion; (M) Bladder; (N) Kidneys; (O) Spine; (P to R) Limbs.

TABLE 3: Minimum requirement checklist at 11–14 weeks scan ISUOG.[2]

Anatomical region	*Minimum requirements*
General	Confirm singleton pregnancy
Head and brain	Axial view of head: • Calcification of cranium • Normal contour/shape with no bony defects • Two brain halves separated by interhemispheric falx • Choroid plexuses filling posterior two-thirds of lateral ventricles ("butterfly sign")
Neck	Sagittal view of head and neck: • Confirm nuchal translucency thickness < 95th centile
Heart	Axial view at four-chamber level: • Heart located inside chest • Regular rhythm
Abdomen	• *Axial view:* Stomach visible • *Abdominal wall intact axial or sagittal view:* Bladder visible and not dilated
Extremities	Four limbs visualized, each with three segments
Placenta	Normal appearance without cystic structures
Biometry	*Sagittal view:* Crown–rump length, nuchal translucency thickness axial view: biparietal diameter

TABLE 4: Anatomical structures that can potentially be visualized on a detailed fetal scan at 11 + 0 to 14 + 0 weeks' gestation (in sagittal, axial or coronal view as needed).[2]

Anatomical region	*Structures to be assessed*
General	Confirmation of singleton pregnancy; overview of fetus, uterus, and placenta
Head and brain	Skull calcification and contour (no bony defects); interhemispheric falx separating cerebral hemispheres; choroid plexus filling posterior two-thirds of lateral ventricles ("butterfly sign"); thalami; brainstem; cerebral peduncles with aqueduct of Sylvius; intracranial translucency (4th ventricle); cisterna magna
Face and neck	Forehead; bilateral orbits; nasal bone; maxilla; retronasal triangle; upper lip; mandible; nuchal translucency thickness; absence of jugular cysts in neck
Thorax	Shape of thoracic wall; lung fields; diaphragmatic continuity
Heart	Cardiac activity with regular rhythm; situs determination; intrathoracic heart position (axis 30–60° to left); heart size ~1/3 of thoracic cavity; four-chamber view with two distinct ventricles (grayscale + color Doppler in diastole); LVOT view (grayscale/color Doppler); three-vessel-and-trachea view (grayscale/color Doppler); absence of tricuspid regurgitation; antegrade ductus venosus A-wave on PW Doppler

Contd...

Contd...

Anatomical region	***Structures to be assessed***
Abdomen	Stomach in the left upper abdomen; bladder normally filled in pelvis (longitudinal diameter <7 mm); intact abdominal wall with normal cord insertion; two umbilical arteries bordering bladder; bilateral kidneys present
Spine	Regular shape and continuity of the vertebral column
Extremities	Upper and lower limbs with three segments each and free movements
Placenta	Normal size and texture (no cystic changes); location in relation to cervix and cesarean scar; cord insertion into placenta
Amniotic fluid and membranes	Amniotic fluid volume appropriate; normal amniotic membrane and chorion dissociation (physiological)

Common Anomalies Detectable at 11–14 Weeks

- *Cranial/Brain:* Anencephaly, acrania, holoprosencephaly, large ventriculomegaly
- *Face/Neck:* Cleft lip, cystic hygroma, increased nuchal translucency
- *Thorax/Heart:* Large defects in cardiac chambers, diaphragmatic hernia (occasionally)
- *Abdomen:* Omphalocele, gastroschisis, megacystis
- *Spine/Skeletal:* Severe scoliosis, limb reduction defects, short-rib dysplasia
- *Others:* Body stalk anomaly, conjoined twins

By applying these structured checklists, the sonographer ensures systematic examination, reducing the risk of missed anomalies and improving reproducibility across centers.

ASSESSMENT OF PLACENTA, CERVIX, AND MATERNAL STRUCTURES

During the first-trimester scan, systematic evaluation should also extend beyond the fetus to include the placenta, cervix, uterus, and adnexa:

- *Placenta:* Echotexture should be reviewed. Abnormal appearances such as masses, cystic spaces, or large subchorionic collections (>5 cm) warrant follow-up. Placental location relative to the cervix is not clinically relevant at this stage, since most low-lying placentas migrate by the mid-trimester. Reporting "placenta previa" in the first trimester is not recommended. In women with a previous caesarean section, special attention should be paid to placental implantation at the scar site, which may indicate caesarean scar pregnancy or placenta accreta spectrum disorders. Early recognition is critical due to the risk of severe complications.

- *Cervix:* Cervical assessment can be performed between 11–14 weeks. Women who deliver preterm often have a shorter cervix at this stage compared with those delivering at term. Correlation exists between first- and second-trimester cervical length measurements. However, there is insufficient evidence to recommend routine cervical length screening in the first trimester until standardized protocols and more outcome data are available.
- *Gynecological pathology:* First-trimester ultrasound may incidentally reveal uterine anomalies (e.g., septate or bicornuate uterus), leiomyomas, or adnexal masses. Both benign and malignant adnexal lesions should be documented when detected.

CONCLUSION

The 11–14 weeks scan is a cornerstone of modern obstetric care, combining accurate dating with early detection of high-risk conditions and fetal anomalies. When performed with standardized protocols and advanced imaging, it provides crucial information for individualized pregnancy management, enabling timely counseling, preventive strategies, and improved maternal–fetal outcomes.

KEY POINTS

- The 11–14 weeks ultrasound is a pivotal scan in modern obstetric care, moving beyond viability and dating to include screening and early anomaly detection.
- Gestational age is most accurately established by crown–rump length (CRL).
- Routine assessment includes confirmation of viability, plurality, chorionicity in multiples, and biometry.
- Aneuploidy risk screening is optimized by combining NT measurement, nasal bone, ductus venosus, and tricuspid flow with maternal serum biochemistry and maternal age.
- Screening for preeclampsia is best performed with the FMF algorithm incorporating maternal risk factors, mean arterial pressure, uterine artery Dopplers, and PlGF.
- A systematic approach using basic and detailed checklists improves the detection of major fetal structural anomalies, with up to two-thirds identifiable in the first trimester.
- Evaluation of the placenta, cervix, uterus, and adnexa provides additional information on maternal and pregnancy complications.

REFERENCES

1. Toms DA. The mechanical index, ultrasound practices, and the ALARA principle. J Ultrasound Med. 2006;25(4):561-2.
2. International Society of Ultrasound in Obstetrics and Gynecology; Bilardo CM, Chaoui R, Hyett JA, Kagan KO, Karim JN,Papageorghiou AT, et al. ISUOG Practice Guidelines (updated): performance of 11–14-week ultrasound scan. Ultrasound Obstet Gynecol. 2023;61:127-43.
3. Hyett JA, Noble PL, Snijders RJ, Montenegro N, Nicolaides KH. Fetal heart rate in trisomy 21 and other chromosomal abnormalities at 10-14 weeks of gestation. Ultrasound Obstet Gynecol. 1996;7(4):239-44.
4. Committee Opinion No 700: Methods for Estimating the Due Date. Obstet Gynecol. 2017;129(5):e150-4.
5. American College of Obstetricians and Gynecologists' Committee on Practice Bulletins—Obstetrics, Committee on Genetics, Society for Maternal-Fetal Medicine. Screening for Fetal Chromosomal Abnormalities: ACOG Practice Bulletin, Number 226. Obstet Gynecol. 2020;136(4):e48–69.
6. Fetal Medicine Foundation. The 11–13+6 weeks scan. London: Fetal Medicine Foundation; [2025]. Available from: https://fetalmedicine.org/fmf/FMF-English.pdf.
7. Cicero S, Rembouskos G, Vandecruys H, Hogg M, Nicolaides KH. Likelihood ratio for trisomy 21 in fetuses with absent nasal bone at the 11-14-week scan. Ultrasound Obstet Gynecol. 2004;23(3):218-23.
8. Maiz N, Valencia C, Kagan KO, Wright D, Nicolaides KH. Ductus venosus Doppler in screening for trisomies 21, 18 and 13 and Turner syndrome at 11-13 weeks of gestation. Ultrasound Obstet Gynecol. 2009;33(5):512-7.
9. Huggon IC, DeFigueiredo DB, Allan LD. Tricuspid regurgitation in the diagnosis of chromosomal anomalies in the fetus at 11-14 weeks of gestation. Heart. 2003;89(9):1071–3.
10. Chaemsaithong P, Sahota DS, Poon LC. First trimester preeclampsia screening and prediction. American Journal of Obstetrics and Gynecology. 2022;226(2):S1071-S1097.e2.

CHAPTER

Ultrasound in Multiple Pregnancies

Uday Thanawala, Priya Deshpande

INTRODUCTION

Ultrasound plays a very important role in multiple pregnancies—from establishing diagnosis to guiding the clinician on how to manage the pregnancy—monitoring growth and health of the fetii—it is an indispensable investigation tool. It helps in decision making in multiple order pregnancies. In this chapter we go through briefly on how to use and interpret ultrasound in mainly twin pregnancies.

Multiple pregnancy is defined as a pregnancy in which a woman is carrying more than one fetus at the same time.

Multiple pregnancy is less common than singleton pregnancy, accounting for about 3 out of every 100 births; twin pregnancies are most frequent, but higher-order multiples do occur.

Causes may include heredity, advanced maternal age, race, and especially the use of ovulation-stimulating medications or assisted reproductive technologies such as IVF **(Figs. 1 to 3).**

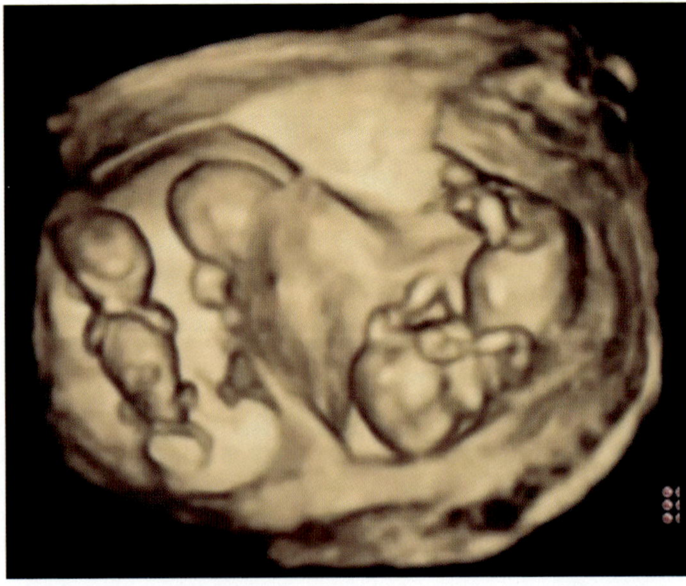

Fig. 1: 3D rendered triplets.

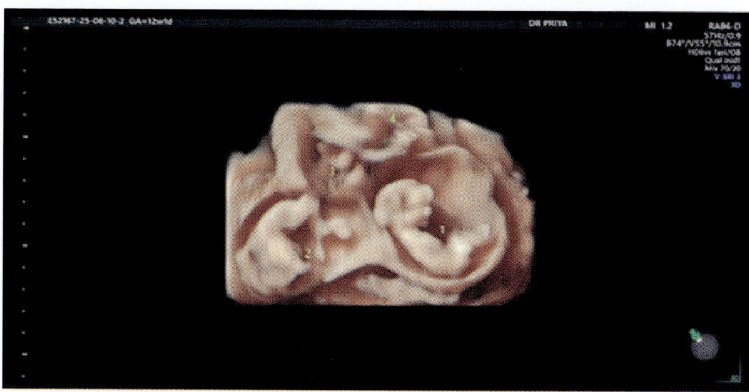

Fig. 2: 3D rendered quadruplets.

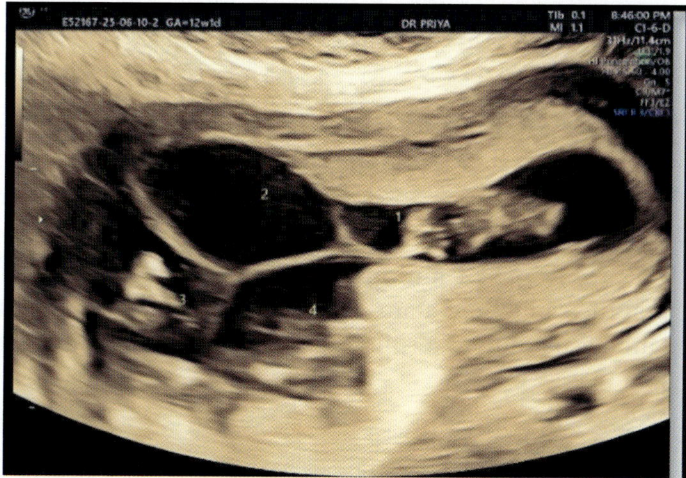

Fig. 3: 2D quadruplets.

Multiple pregnancy usually refers to:

- *Twins:* Two fetuses
- *Triplets:* Three fetuses
- *Quadruplets:* Four fetuses
- *Quintuplets:* Five fetuses
- *Sextuplets:* Six fetuses
- *Septuplets:* Seven fetuses

Multiple pregnancy can occur naturally or as a result of fertility treatments, and the fetuses may be:

- *Monozygotic:* Arising from a single fertilized egg that splits into two or more embryos. These fetuses are genetically identical and always the same sex.
- *Dizygotic:* Resulting from two or more separate eggs fertilized by different sperm. These fetuses are genetically distinct, like ordinary siblings, and can be the same or different sexes.

Multiple pregnancies, spontaneous or assisted, invite multiple troubles as there is a high risk of complications, more so in monochorionicity, higher maternal and fetal risks, needs more frequent ultrasound monitoring and tailored antenatal care and delivery planning.

DETECTION OF MULTIPLE PREGNANCY

When?

- Better identified in the first trimester between 6–12 weeks of gestation
- Accuracy is >95% at first trimester (11–13.6 weeks).[1]

How?

Transvaginal scan preferably for clear visualization of the membranes and accurate results.

Key Findings on Ultrasound

Number of gestational sacs corresponds to chronicity.

Triplets

Triplets refer to a type of multiple pregnancy involving three fetuses developing at the same time. Rare-1 in 10,000 pregnancies naturally[2]—but the rate is increasing due to fertility treatments and assisted reproductive technologies.

Types of Triplets

- Trichorionic triamniotic triplets
- Dichorionic triamniotic triplets with one monochorionic pair
- Higher order than triplets occur rarely and the principles of labeling remain as in twins and triplets.

Labeling of Twins on Ultrasound

Importance of Accurate Labeling

- *Continuity of care:* Ensures correct identification of each fetus across serial scans and providers, reducing the interobserver variation.
- *Tracking anomalies or growth discrepancies:* Especially vital in cases of selective growth restriction or congenital anomalies.
- *Critical for selective fetal reduction or invasive procedures* (e.g., amniocentesis, laser therapy).
- *Avoids wrong-fetus interventions:* A serious clinical and medicolegal issue.

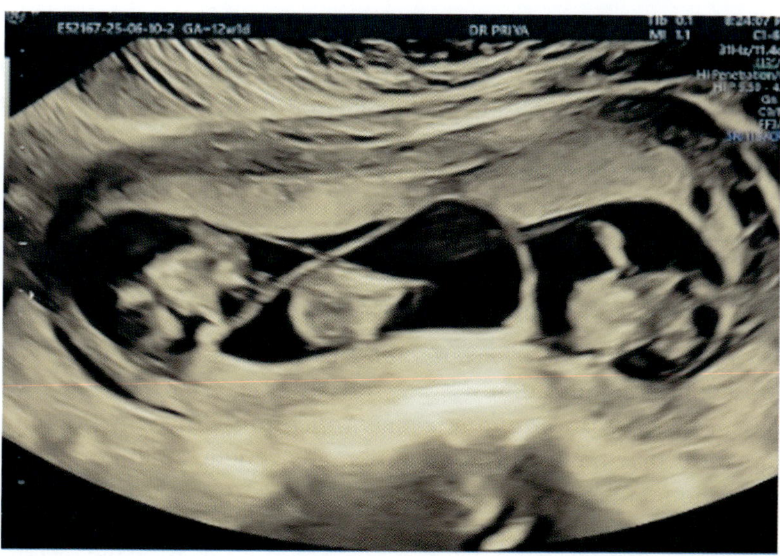

Fig. 4: 2D triplets.

Methods of Twin Labeling

- Twin 1 = fetus/gestational sac *closest to the internal os or cervix* (presenting fetus).
- Twin 2 = fetus/gestational sac *higher in the uterus* (non-presenting).

This system is used in first trimester and is generally maintained throughout unless delivery order changes due to malpresentation.

- *Left/Right orientation:* Based on *maternal anatomical left/right* when fetus position is ambiguous.
- *Superior/Inferior:* Especially used when both fetuses are transverse.

Biometric and Placental Landmarks

- Chorionicity helps anchor labeling:
  - In dichorionic twins, the fetus corresponding to a specific placenta is tracked.
  - For *monochorionic twins*, biometric differences or cord insertion positions may help.
  - Keep a *"fetal map"* in the chart with placental assignment and biometric data **(Fig. 4)**.

Once diagnosed it is important to label the fetuses for proper follow-up. In today's date generally physicians and patients both would possibly not opt for more than twins—thus fetal reduction is an important intervention.

Higher order pregnancies generally would opt for fetal reduction and bring down the number to twins.

SELECTIVE FETAL REDUCTION

Selective fetal reduction (SFR) is a procedure used to reduce the number of fetuses in a multiple pregnancy, typically performed to improve maternal and perinatal outcomes.

It has important clinical, ethical, and psychosocial considerations. Proper counselling is a must and the patient must understand that any intervention has its risks.

Indications for Selective Fetal Reduction

- *High-order multiples (triplets or more), can occur especially with IVF/ART:* Most common indication
- *Discordant fetal anomalies or complications:* In twin pregnancies, one fetus may have a structural anomaly, genetic condition, or growth restriction.
- *Monochorionic complications:* For example, Twin-Twin Transfusion Syndrome (TTTS), Selective Intrauterine Growth Restriction (sIUGR), TRAP sequence.

Techniques of Reduction

Depends on chorionicity:

- *Dichorionic twins:* Intracardiac potassium chloride (KCl) injection.
- *Monochorionic twins:* Cord occlusion methods (e.g., bipolar coagulation, radiofrequency ablation, laser ablation, microwave ablation), since KCl can affect the co-twin via vascular connections.

Timing

Usually performed between 11–14 weeks, but can be done later if anomaly/ aneuploidy is detected late.

Advantages of Selective Fetal Reduction

Maternal and perinatal outcomes:

- Improved survival and outcomes in the remaining fetus(es) compared to continuation of high-order pregnancy.
- Reduced risks of preterm birth, low birth weight, and preeclampsia.

Procedure-related loss rates:

- Vary with technique, timing, chorionicity, operator experience, and skills.
- Typically it is 5–10% in monochorionic twins; <5% in dichorionic twins.[3]
- Outcomes in late selective fetal reduction due to fetal anomaly may depend on gestational age and chorionicity.

Ethical and Psychological Aspects

- Ethical dilemmas arise, particularly in reducing from twins to singleton.
- Psychological impact on parents can be significant—feelings of grief or guilt.
- Counseling plays a key role pre- and post-procedure.

Guidelines and Recommendations

- ISUOG (International Society of Ultrasound in Obstetrics and Gynecology): Provides guidance on when and how to perform SFR.
- ACOG and RCOG also emphasize multidisciplinary care and individualized decision-making.
- Informed consent is critical, with discussion of risks, benefits, alternatives, and emotional implications.

TWINS

Dichorionic Diamniotic DCDA Twins

- Two gestational sacs seen as fluid filled structures seen around 4.5-5 weeks, with a fairly thick intervening membrane and the lambda sign at the insertion of the membrane
- Two yolk sacs seen around 5 weeks onwards
- Two embryos visualized around 6 weeks onwards with cardiac activity **(Figs. 5 to 10)**.
- Two separate placentas—anterior and posterior; on the same side with lambda sign **(Fig. 11)**

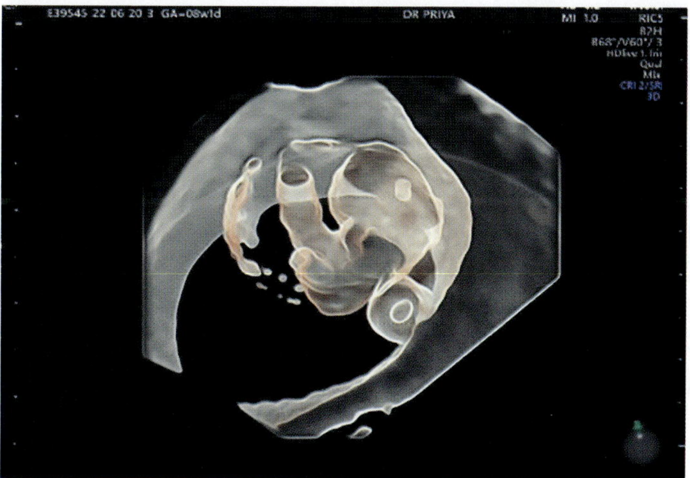

Fig. 5: Embryo and yolk sac in 3D silhouette render.

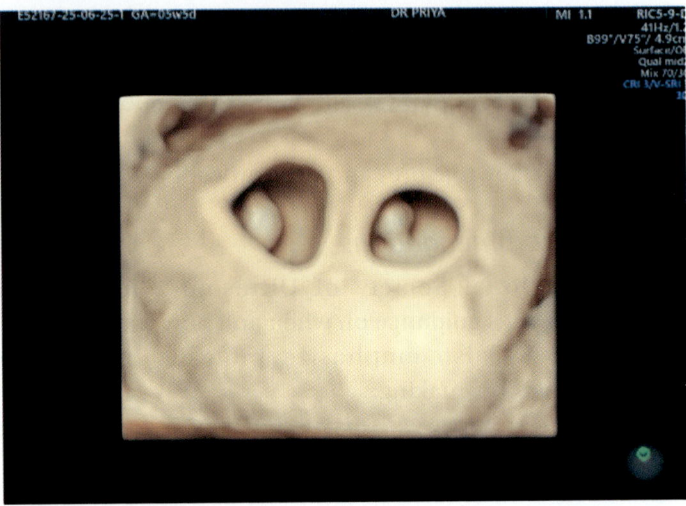

Fig. 6: 3D rendered early pregnancy twins with 2 gestational sacs and yolk sacs.

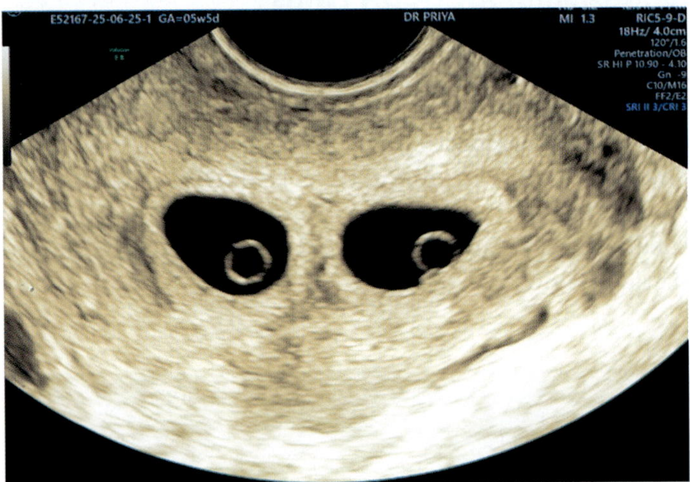

Fig. 7: 2D early pregnancy dichorionic twins with 2 gestational sacs and 2 yolk sacs.

Lambda sign is seen as there is chorionic tissue protruding between the amniotic membranes in dichorionic pregnancies.

Monochorionic Diamniotic MCDA Twins

One gestational sac with two yolk sacs/two embryos.

Monochorionic Monoamniotic MCMA Twins

One gestational sac, one or two yolk sac, one amniotic membrane and two embryos.

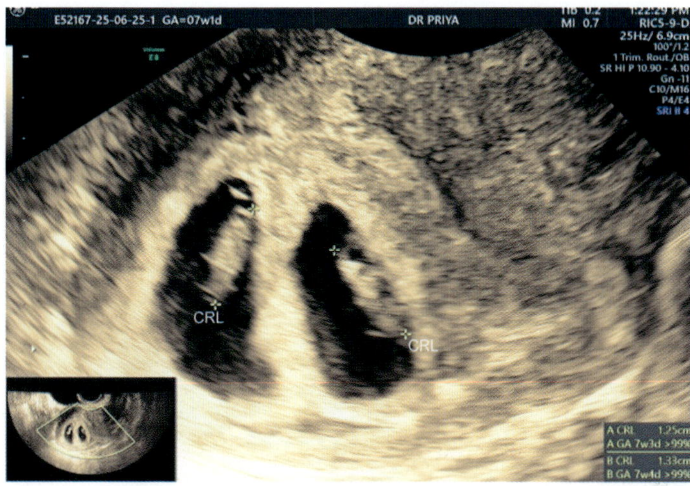

Fig. 8: 2 D dichorionic twins with 2 embryos.

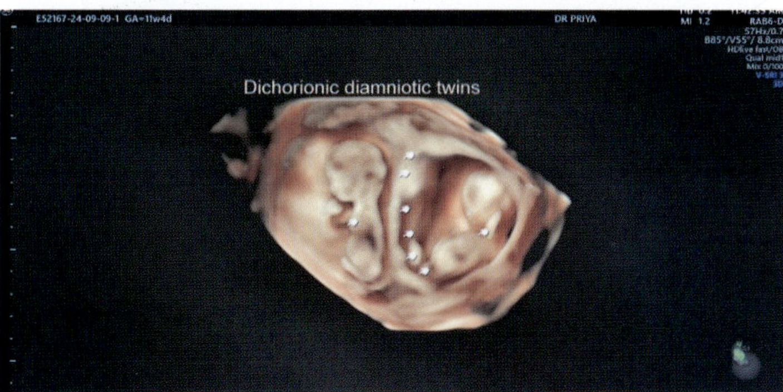

Fig. 9: 3D rendered dichorionic twins and silhouette rendered mode.

To be doubly sure, transvaginal assessment with increasing the gain settings should be done to visualize the membrane if present; as it can be very thin and hence easily missed transabdominally **(Fig. 12).**

T sign in monochorionic twin pregnancies.

WHY DETERMINING CHORIONICITY IS MOST CRUCIAL?

Any ultrasound reporting of twin pregnancy is incomplete without determining and reporting chorionicity.

Monochorionic twins have shared placenta—increased risk of TTTS, selective FGR/growth discordance.

Dichorionic twins have separate placentas and hence lower risk of such complications **(Table 1)**.

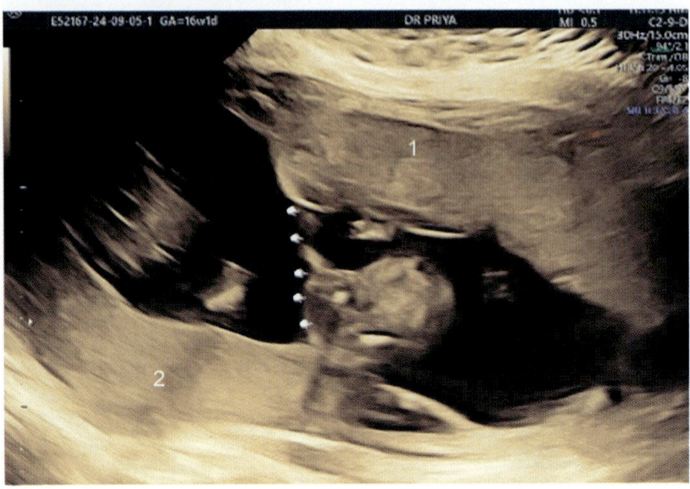

Fig. 10: Two separate placentas of dichorionic twins.

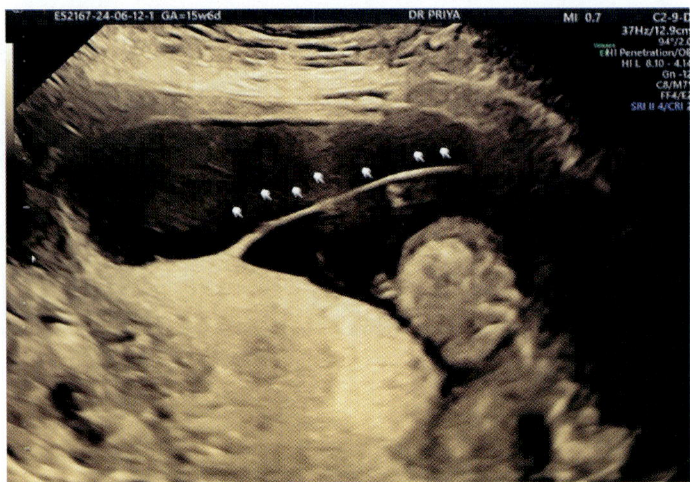

Fig. 11: Lambda sign in dichorionic twins.

FIRST TRIMESTER SCREENING—NT SCAN

Done between 11–13.6 weeks of gestation with the CRL that corresponds to 45–84 mm.

Ultrasound markers are:

1. Nuchal translucency NT
2. Nasal bone
3. Tricuspid Doppler flow
4. Ductus venosus Doppler

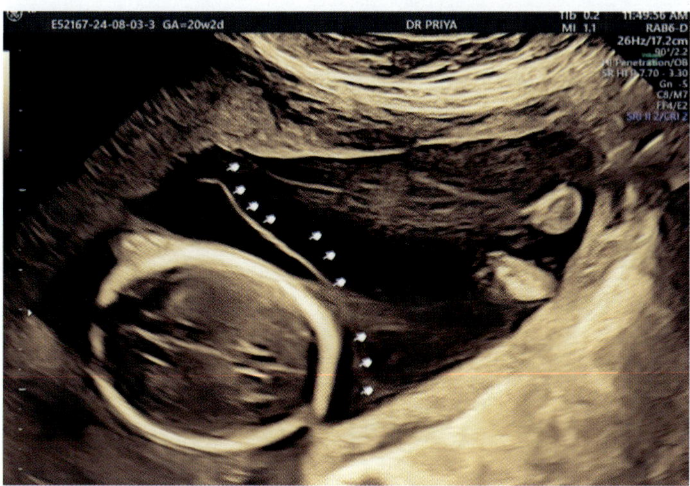

Fig. 12: T sign in monochorionic twins.

TABLE 1: Ultrasound markers for chorionicity.

Key ultrasound markers		
Features	***Dichorionic***	***Monochorionic***
Number of placentas	2 (may fuse)	1
Membrane thickness	>2 mm (thick)	<2 mm (thin)
Lambda sign (Twin peak sign)	Present	Absent
T sign	Absent	Present
Sex of fetuses (at later gestation)	Can be different/same	Same

5. Structural assessment for major anomalies
6. Uterine artery Doppler study to screen for preeclampsia **(Figs. 13 to 17)**

SERUM BIOCHEMISTRY AND ITS ROLE IN TWIN GESTATION

1. Papp A
2. Serum free beta-hCG

Risk assessment is as per fetus in DCDA twins and for the pregnancy in MCDA twins.

However, in a twin pregnancy, this assessment becomes less straightforward for two main reasons:

- *Masking effect:* If only one of the two fetuses has a chromosomal abnormality, the normal hormone levels produced by the unaffected twin can "mask" or average out the abnormal levels from the affected twin. This can lead to a false-negative result, where the test incorrectly shows a low risk.

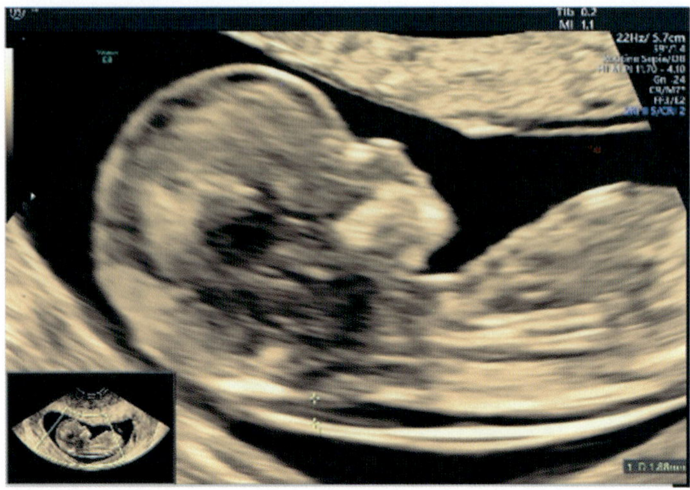

Fig. 13: NT image.

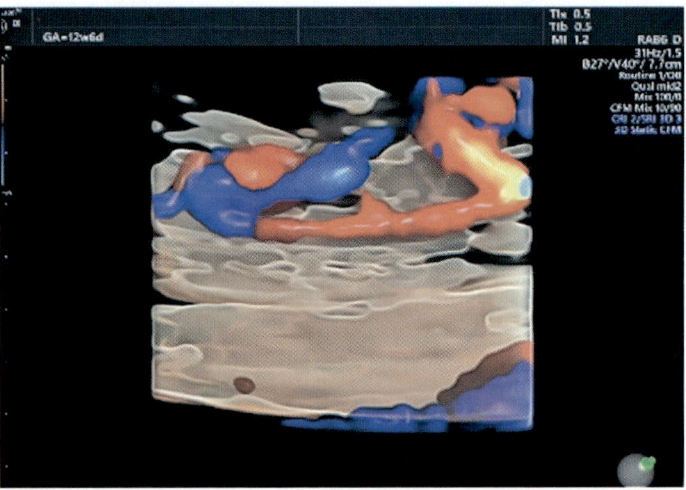

Fig. 14: Fetal circulation 3D rendered.

- *Altered marker levels:* Twin pregnancies naturally have different (usually higher) levels of pregnancy-related hormones in the mother's blood compared to singleton pregnancies. This makes it difficult to interpret the results and apply standard risk calculations.[4]

The detection rates are less and sensitivity also varies depending on whether the twins are monozygotic) or dizygotic.[5] Hence, in multiple pregnancies alternative screening methods, such as Non-invasive prenatal testing (NIPT) which has shown higher sensitivity in detecting Down syndrome is opted.

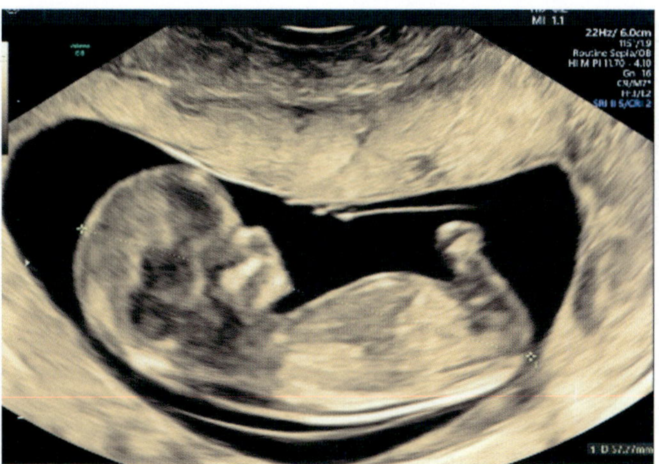

Fig. 15: Crown–rump length in first trimester.

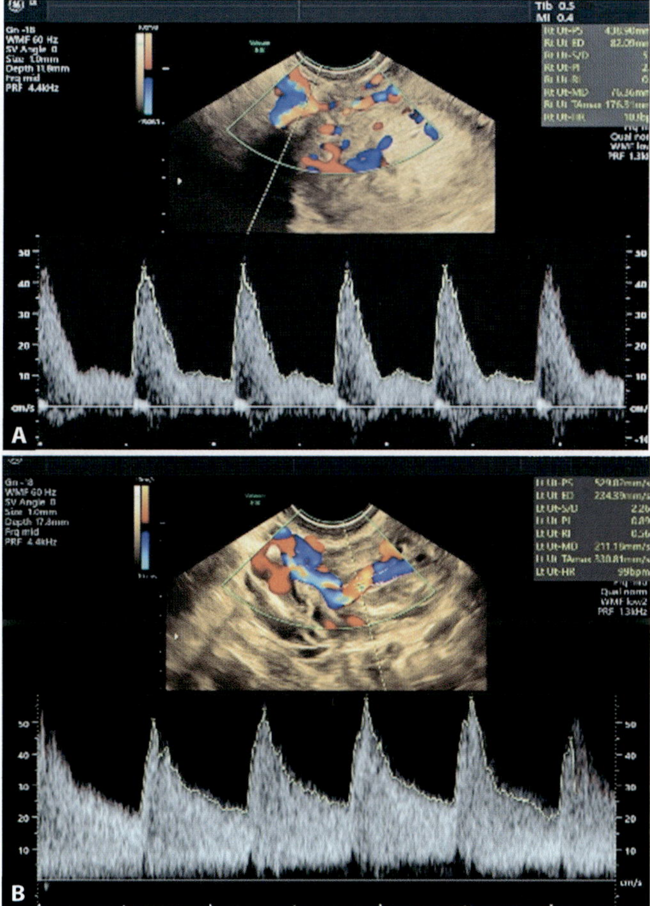

Figs. 16A and B: Right and left uterine artery Doppler.

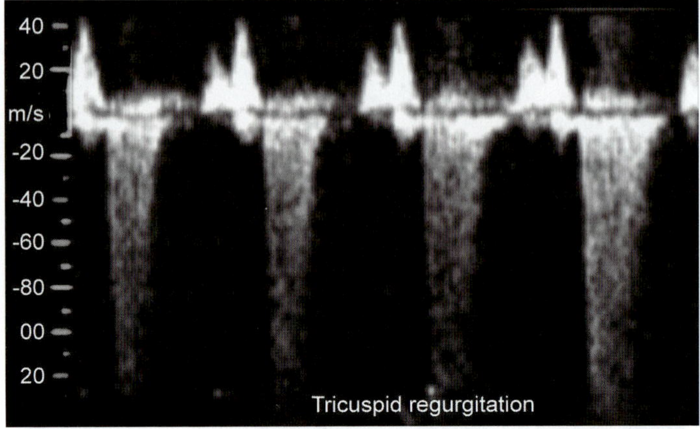

Fig. 17: Tricuspid Doppler showing regurgitation.

CELL FREE FETAL DNA (NIPT) IN TWINS

- Can be offered from 10 weeks onwards.
- According to the ISUOG practice guidelines 2025; NIPT is the most accurate screening test for trisomy 21 with detection rate of 99% and false positive rate of 0.02%.[6,7]
- SNP based NIPT platforms can determine zygosity and assign individual fetal fractions.
- Contraindications—vanishing twin, as the dead fetus can contribute to the cell free DNA in maternal circulation for few weeks (6–8 weeks) its demise.
- Thorough pre-test and post-test counseling is a MUST.

If NIPT comes positive for chromosomal defect—amniocentesis—which sac?

In twins; it is prudent to test both sacs even if the fetii appears normal.

VANISHING TWIN

Refers to spontaneous demise and resorption of one of the twins in multiple gestation.

Incidence—10–30% in early twin pregnancies.

Ultrasound is the best modality for screening in surviving twin such cases. Biochemical markers can be altered hence serum screening should be avoided—especially when there is a measurable CRL of the vanishing twin.[8,9]

cfDNA from the demised twin can persist in maternal blood for weeks leading to false positive results/no call rates in NIPT.

The surviving fetus then undergoes regular antenatal care.

At this early stage there is NO risk of any effect on the surviving fetus or coagulation disorder in the mother.

SECOND TRIMESTER SCREENING/ANOMALY SCAN

When?

18–22 weeks gestation.

Labeling of Twins

- Twin A: Closer to cervix
- Twin B: Higher position

Objectives

1. Detect fetal anomalies
2. Confirm chorionicity and amnionicity (if not confirmed previously)
3. Assess amniotic fluid in each sac
4. Evaluate placental location and number
5. Cervical assessment (transvaginally for accurate measurement)

Challenges in Twin Anomaly Scan

- Overlapping fetal parts
- Thin intertwin membrane
- Confusion in identification and labeling (use landmarks like placental location, fetal position and mention in each report to avoid interobserver variation)
- Limited views in later gestation.

CERVICAL LENGTH ASSESSMENT

- At the anomaly scan—a cervical length of less than 2.5 cm is regarded as a cut off and high risk of preterm delivery.
- In twins and higher order pregnancies one does not have data to set a cut off—but if the cervix is short (<2.5 cm) on anomaly scan—the risk could be high for preterm and some measures like: Progesterone or Tightening of Os need to be considered.[10,11]

Congenital Anomalies? Discordant Anomaly

Risk of birth defects doubles compared to singleton pregnancies.

Case

Dichorionic diamniotic twin pregnancy; one twin had acrania and other twin was normal at NT scan suggestive of discordant anomaly. Selective fetal reduction of the twin with acrania was opted for **(Figs. 18 to 21)**.

USG FOR MONITORING GROWTH OF TWINS

General Guideline

Suggested timing of USG in twins gestation shown in **Table 2**.

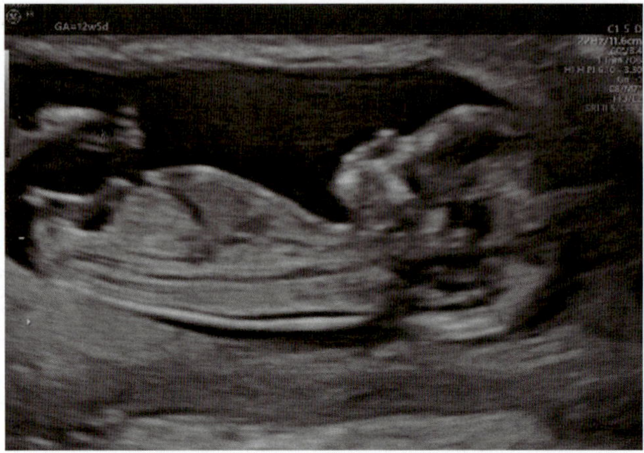

Fig. 18: Dichorionic twin with one normal twin.

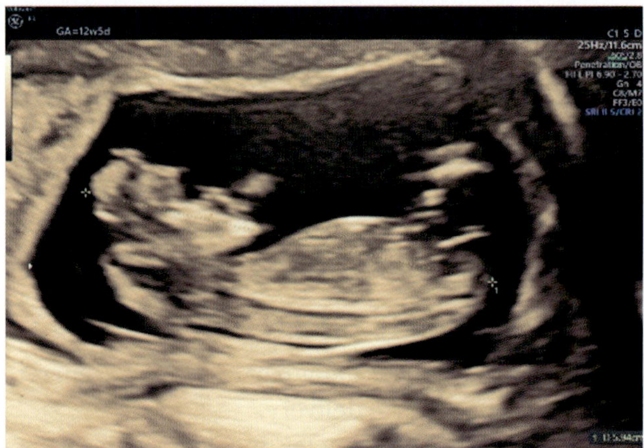

Fig. 19: Acrania.

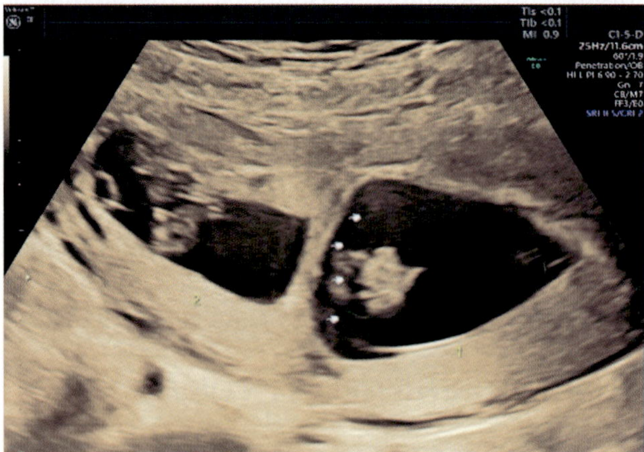

Fig. 20: Two gestational sacs.

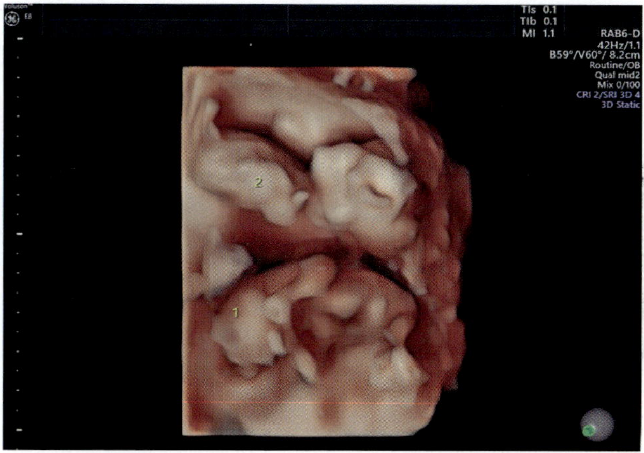

Fig. 21: 3D rendered dichorionic twins.

TABLE 2: Suggested timing of USG in twins gestation.

Feature	*DCDA twins*	*MCDA twins*
Ultrasound monitoring	Every 4 weeks 20 weeks onwards	Every 2 weeks 16 weeks onwards
Anomaly scan	19–20 weeks	19–20 weeks
Delivery	37–38 weeks	32–34 weeks

Growth and Doppler Assessment[12]

- Every 2 weeks for MCDA twins
- Every 4 weeks for DCDA twins.

Chart the growth to assess the growth velocity on standard growth charts.

If one fetus now shows a major anomaly then the option for fetal reduction can still be offered to the patient.

Growth Discordance

$$\frac{\text{Estimated Fetal Weight (EFW) of larger twin} - \text{EFW of smaller twin}}{\text{EFW of larger twin}} \times 100$$

>20–25% discordance is significant.

Amniotic Fluid Assessment

Deepest vertical pocket/Maximum vertical pocket in each sac.

DOPPLER ASSESSMENT

- *Umbilical artery Doppler:* 16 weeks onwards in MCDA twins and 20 weeks onwards in DCDA twins

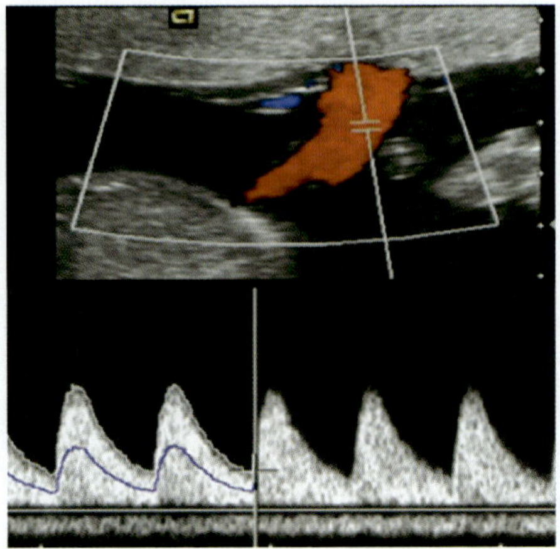

Fig. 22: Increased resistance in umbilical artery Doppler in Type I sFGR.

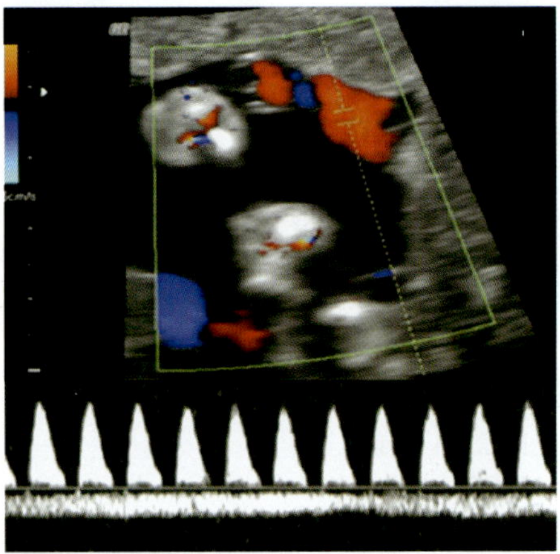

Fig. 23: Absent end diastolic flow in umbilical artery Doppler Type II sFGR.

- *Middle cerebral artery Doppler:* 20 weeks onwards in MCDA and MCMA twins for twin anemia polycythemia sequence (TAPS) screening.

Once there is significant growth discordance—it is imperative to follow up these fetii with umbilical and MCA Doppler studies frequently—the growth restricted twin may show absent diastolic flow and a Ductus Venosus doppler may be needed to be watched closely if one needs to gain more time for lung maturity.[13,14]

Types of Doppler changes in Growth Restricted Fetus:

- *Type I:* Umbilical artery doppler end diastolic flow positive
- *Type II:* Umbilical artery Doppler EDF absent or reversed
- *Type III:* Umbilical artery Doppler EDF cyclical change from positive to absent and reversed **(Figs. 22 to 24)**

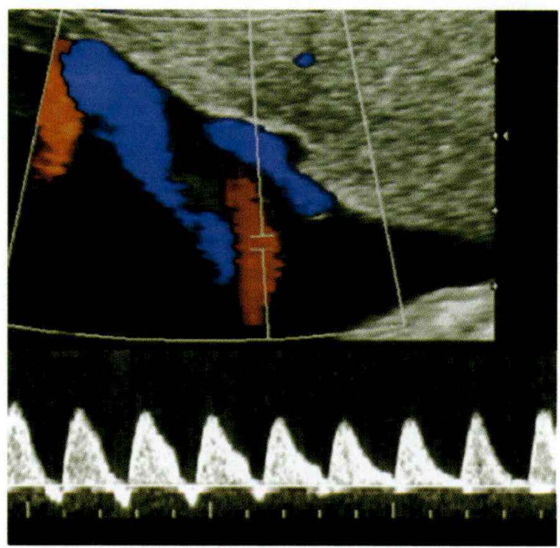

Fig. 24: Cyclical reversed and positive end diastolic flow Type III sFGR.

TABLE 3: Quintero classification.[17]

Quintero stage	*Sonographic or Doppler findings*
I	Polyhydramnios, DVP ≥8 cm in recipient's sac and oligohydramnios, DVP ≤2 cm in donor's sac with visible bladder in donor
II	As in Stage I but no visible bladder in donor
III	As in Stage II and abnormal Doppler flow of umbilical artery, umbilical vein or ductus venosus
IV	As in Stage III and hydrops of either twin
V	Fetal demise of one or both twins

COMPLICATIONS IN MONOCHORIONIC TWIN PREGNANCY

Twin-to-Twin Transfusion Syndrome (TTTS)

A condition specific to monochorionic (placenta-sharing) twins, involving abnormal blood vessel connections—*large central arterio-venous connections* and imbalanced blood flow between twins. This can cause significant morbidity and mortality.

Incidence: 10:15%

Due to abnormal sharing of blood between twins via placental blood vessels-arterial-venous anastomosis leading to one twin being overloaded with blood affecting fluid volumes and growth **(Tables 3 and 4)**.

Laser Photocoagulation

This is the therapy option, where laser is used to ablate the anastomosing blood vessels and effectively cause dichorionization of the placenta; separating the circulations by cutting off the connections causing the TTTS

TABLE 4: Quintero stages and suggested treatment.

Stage	*Features*	*Treatment*
I	Oligohydramnios with deepest vertical pocket (DVP) <2 cm in donor sac and polyhydramnios in the recipient sac (DVP) >8 cm	Conservative
II	Bladder of the donor twin not visible	
III	Doppler studies are critically abnormal in either the donor or recipient	Laser photocoagulation <26 weeks
IV	Hydrops present usually in the recipient	
V	One or both babies have died (not amenable to therapy)	

TABLE 5: Staging for TAPS.[18]

Criteria for diagnosis and staging:	
Stage 1	> 0.5 Mom difference in delta MCA PSV
Stage 2	> 0.7 Mom difference in delta MCA PSV
Stage 3	Stage 1/2 with cardiac compromise of the donor
Stage 4	Donor develops hydrops
Stage 5	One or both babies IUFD

Twin Anemia-Polycythemia Sequence (TAPS)

A rare complication where chronic blood transfer due to *tiny peripheral artery-venous connections*; leads to one twin being anemic and the other polycythemic **(Table 5)**.

It can cause intrauterine fetal demise, brain damage, limb necrosis.

Twin Reversed Arterial Perfusion (TRAP) Sequence

- Rare; one twin develops without a functioning heart and is dependent on the other for circulation
- TRAP is seen in 2.5% of monochorionic twin pregnancies
- More common in monoamniotic than diamniotic monochorionic twins
- 33% mortality—1st and early 2nd trimester
- Causes of mortality are cardiac failure and polyhydramnios
- Prophylactic treatment before 16 weeks—debatable-TRAPIST TRIAL
- Invasive treatment modalities are interstitial laser or radiofrequency ablation and coagulation of fetal vessels or endoscopic ablation of fetal blood vessels
- Post treatment survival rate is 75–80%.

MONOCHORIONIC MONOAMNIOTIC TWIN PREGNANCY

Two weekly scans; 16 weeks onwards to assess fetal growth and Doppler to screen for TAPS and selective FGR.

20 weeks onwards twice weekly scan to assess for cord entanglement **(Figs. 25 and 26)**.

Delivery timing at 32–34 weeks as the risk of complications is high in MCMA twins.

Amniotic Fluid Imbalance

Both excessive (polyhydramnios) and reduced (oligohydramnios) amniotic fluid levels are more common, usually linked to placental discordance or TTTS.

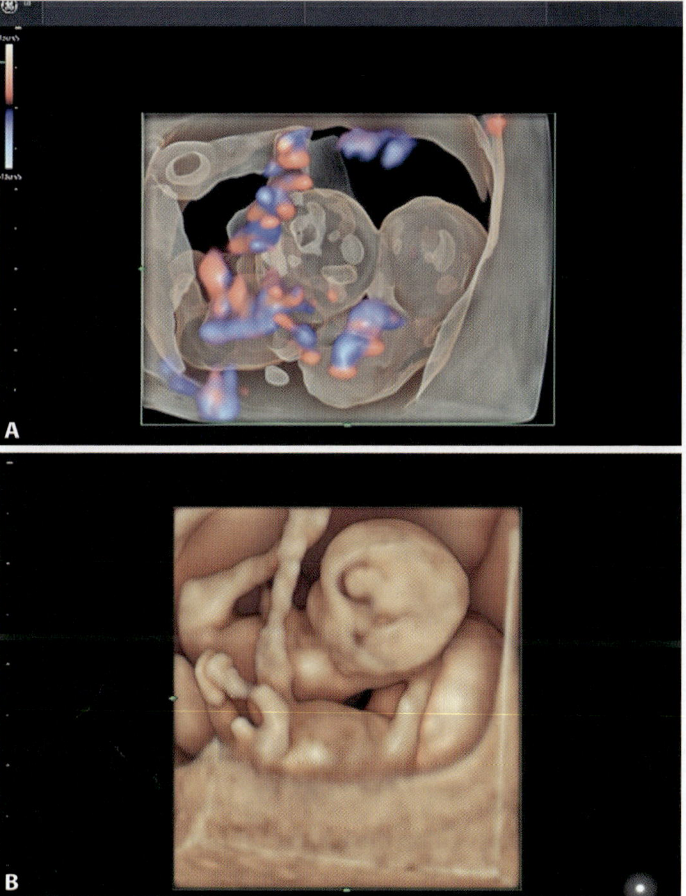

Figs. 25A and B: 3D rendered monochorionic monoamniotic twins.

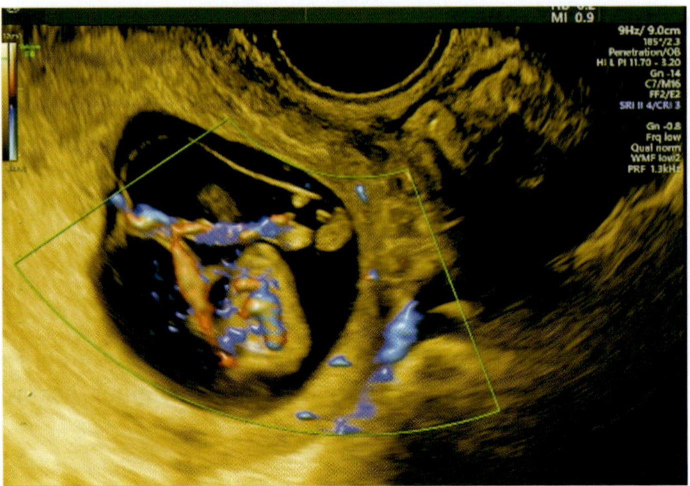

Fig. 26: Color Doppler demonstration of the umbilical arteries in monoamniotic twins.

Miscarriage and Fetal Loss

- Increased risk of losing one or both fetuses, with "vanishing twin syndrome" referring to the loss of one fetus early in pregnancy i.e., <14 weeks gestation
- *Loss of one twin:* IUFD can happen in complications like TTTS, selective FGR, TRAP in monochorionic twin pregnancies due to intra placental arterio-arterial and arterio-venous avascular anastomosis.

In Case of IUFD in Later Gestation

In DADC twins: The surviving twin can have a normal growth and outcome and the risk to mother is minimal in terms of coagulation disorder.

In monochorionic twins there is a possibility of cerebral damage to the surviving twin, due to sudden fall in the blood pressure of the demised twin. Sometimes, there is fetal anemia in the surviving twin due to sudden blood loss and may need rescue blood transfusion.

The surviving fetus needs regular ultrasound monitoring of fetal brain in particular and fetal MRI brain can also be a useful assisting tool to diagnose ischemic damage to the surviving fetus.

CONCLUSION

A multiple pregnancy requires close medical supervision given the increased maternal and fetal risks. Regular ultrasound monitoring, is important to guide the clinician. Towards delivery time ultrasound gives is important information about the position and expected weight of the babies to plan a safe delivery.

REFERENCES

1. Khalil, A., Sotiriadis, A., Baschat, A., Bhide, A., Gratacós, E., Hecher, K., Lewi, L., Salomon, L.J., Thilaganathan, B. and Ville, Y. (2025), ISUOG Practice Guidelines (updated): role of ultrasound in twin pregnancy. Ultrasound Obstet Gynecol, 65: 253-276. https://doi.org/10.1002/uog.29166
2. ISUOG Practice Guidelines: role of ultrasound in twin pregnancy Ultrasound Obstet Gynecol. 2016;47:247–263. DOI: 10.1002/uog.15821
3. pubmed.ncbi.nlm.nih.gov/8821849 Multiple marker screening for Down syndrome in twin pregnancies
4. Dias T, Mahsud-Dornan S, Thilaganathan B, Papageorghiou A, Bhide A. First-trimester ultrasound dating of twin pregnancy: are singleton charts reliable? BJOG 2010;117:979–984.
5. DeYoung TH, Stortz SK, Riffenburgh RH, et al. Establishing the most accurate due date in dichorionic twin gestations by first and second trimester ultrasound. J Ultrasound Med. 2021;40(11):2319-2327.
6. Southwest Thames Obstetric Research Collaborative (STORK). Prospective risk of late stillbirth in monochorionic twins: a regional cohort study. Ultrasound Obstet Gynecol. 2012;39(5):500-504.
7. Seong JS, Han YJ, Kim MH, et al. The risk of preterm birth in vanishing twin: a multicenter prospective cohort study. PLoS One. 2020;15(5):1-9.
8. Kagan KO, Gazzoni A, Sepulveda-Gonzalez G, Sotiriadis A, Nicolaides KH. Discordance in nuchal translucency thickness in the prediction of severe twin-to-twin transfusion syndrome. Ultrasound Obstet Gynecol. 2007;29:527–532.
9. D'Antonio F, Khalil A, Dias T, Thilaganathan B; Southwest Thames Obstetric Research Collaborative. Crown–rump length discordance and adverse perinatal outcome in twins: analysis of the Southwest Thames Obstetric Research Collaborative (STORK) multiple pregnancy cohort. Ultrasound Obstet Gynecol 2013;41:621–626.
10. D'Antonio F, Khalil A, Pagani G, Papageorghiou AT, Bhide A, Thilaganathan B. Crown–rump length discordance and adverse perinatal outcome in twin pregnancies: systematic review and meta-analysis. Ultrasound Obstet Gynecol. 2014;44:138–146.
11. Salomon LJ, Alfirevic Z, Bilardo CM, Chalouhi GE, Ghi T, Kagan KO, Lau TK, Papageorghiou AT, Raine-Fenning NJ, Stirnemann J, Suresh S, Tabor A, Timor-Tritsch IE, Toi A, Yeo G. ISUOG practice guidelines: performance of first-trimester fetal ultrasound scan. Ultrasound Obstet Gynecol. 2013;41:102–113.
12. Rossi AC, D'Addario V. Umbilical cord occlusion for selective feticide in complicated monochorionic twins: a systematic review of literature. Am J Obstet Gynecol. 2009;200:123–129.
13. Conde-Agudelo A, Romero R. Prediction of preterm birth in twin gestations using biophysical and biochemical tests. Am J Obstet Gynecol. 2014;211:583–595.
14. Stirrup OT, Khalil A, D'Antonio F, Thilaganathan B, on behalf of the Southwest Thames Obstetric Research Collaborative (STORK). Fetal growth reference ranges in twin pregnancy: analysis of the Southwest Thames Obstetric Research Collaborative (STORK) multiple pregnancy cohort. Ultrasound Obstet Gynecol. 2015;45:301–307.
15. Nakata M, Sumie M, Murata S, Miwa I, Kusaka E, Sugino N. A case of monochorionic twin pregnancy complicated with intrauterine single fetal death with successful

treatment of intrauterine blood transfusion in the surviving fetus. Fetal Diagn Ther. 2007;22:7–9.

16. Slaghekke F, Kist WJ, Oepkes D, Pasman SA, Middeldorp JM, Klumper FJ, Walther FJ, Vandenbussche FP, Lopriore E. Twin anemia-polycythemia sequence: diagnostic criteria, classification, perinatal management and outcome. Fetal Diagn Ther. 2010;27:181–190.
17. Chalouhi GE, Marangoni MA, Quibel T, Deloison B, Benzina N, Essaoui M, Al Ibrahim A, Stirnemann JJ, Salomon LJ, Ville Y. Active management of selective intrauterine growth restriction with abnormal Doppler in monochorionic diamniotic twin pregnancies diagnosed in the second trimester of pregnancy. Prenat Diagn. 2013;33:109–115.
18. Weitzner O, Barrett J, Murphy KE, Kingdom J, Aviram A, Mei-Dan E, Hiersch L, Ryan G, Van Mieghem T, Abbasi N, Fox NS, Rebarber A, Berghella V, Melamed N. National and international guidelines on the management of twin pregnancies: a comparative review. Am J Obstet Gynecol. 2023;229(6):577-598. doi: 10.1016/j.ajog.2023.05.022. Epub 2023 May 25. PMID: 37244456.

5 CHAPTER

Ultrasound in Third Trimester

Vandana Bansal, Rupal Parekh

BACKGROUND

The main objective of third trimester obstetrical ultrasound examination is to provide accurate diagnostic information regarding fetal growth (both growth restriction and macrosomia) and Doppler flows, fetal wellbeing, amniotic fluid volume, fetal presentation, placental localization and cord insertion and may also be used as a second look for various late onset fetal anomalies.

The rationale is to identify and triage risk pregnancies and improve outcomes via timely management. This is not solely possible by clinical examination alone. It helps in reducing maternal and neonatal morbidity and mortality by timely diagnosis, timely decisions and interventions and better postnatal preparedness towards managing early neonatal problems.

CURRENT SCENARIO OF OBSTETRIC IMAGING IN INDIA AND THE WORLD

It is universally recommended that all high-risk pregnancies should be offered serial ultrasound for growth assessment from 26–28 weeks of gestation. Additionally, third trimester scan is used selectively in late pregnancy where there are specific clinical indications. Routine late pregnancy ultrasound screening in unselected low-risk population is currently not recommended by most guidelines due to insufficient evidence of its benefit and the lack of cost effectiveness in resource constrain settings. However more and more recent studies have shown that routine third trimester ultrasonography, including Doppler, can help in risk-stratification of otherwise clinically low-risk pregnancies and improve perinatal survival.

The Ministry of Health and Family welfare government of India has published guidelines on the use of ultrasonography during pregnancy which recommend only one obstetric ultrasound during pregnancy between 18 and 19 weeks of pregnancy as part of routine Ante Natal Care (ANC) package which provides opportunity to diagnose congenital anomalies and detect soft markers of aneuploidy. This single scan will also give information on gestational age and number of live fetuses with placental location and pelvic pathology if any. Additional ultrasound examinations can be done if clinically indicated. There is no mention of a third trimester ultrasound in our Indian guidelines.[1]

WHO recommendations on antenatal care for a positive pregnancy experience (2016) states one ultrasound scan before 24 weeks should be done for pregnant women to estimate gestational age, improve detection of fetal anomalies and multiple pregnancies, reduce number of inductions for post term pregnancy and improve a woman's pregnancy experience. No routine doppler ultrasound examination in the third trimester nor any late pregnancy scan is recommended.[2]

Hence the need for any additional third-trimester scans is based on local guidelines, clinical requirement and presence of maternal or fetal risk factors that are known to be associated with abnormal growth.

INDICATIONS/COMPONENTS OF ULTRASOUND EXAMINATION IN THIRD TRIMESTER

A standard list of indications for which a second or third trimester ultrasound may be asked for has been enumerated by the AIUM ACR ACOG SMFM SRU guidelines on Practice parameters for performance of standard diagnostic ultrasound examination, 2018.[3] These may be indicated at any time even in the third trimester as per the clinical situation. The starred indications may not be accurately determined in the third trimester and are more accurate in the second trimester but in developing countries like ours, this may be the first time that the patient may report for ultrasound.

Standard Second and Third Trimester USG Examination[3]

1. *Estimate gestational age**
2. *Number of feti and chorionicity**
3. Identify fetal presentation and placental location
4. Evaluation of fetal anatomy and follow-up screening for the anomalies*
5. Assessment of cervical length
6. Assess fetal wellbeing with fetal growth and color doppler.
7. Evaluation of a significant discrepancy between uterine size and clinical gestational age, poor maternal weight gain
8. Suspected amniotic fluid abnormalities
9. Evaluation of premature rupture of membranes and/or preterm labor
10. Evaluation of vaginal bleeding
11. Evaluation of abdominal or pelvic pain
12. Suspected placental abruption in antepartum bleeding
13. Evaluation of placental pathology such as placenta previa and morbidly adherent placenta spectrum
14. Suspected fetal death for viability
15. Adjunct to amniocentesis, CVS, fetal reduction or other invasive procedure
16. Adjunct to maneuver such as external cephalic version

17. Evaluation of a pelvic mass*
18. Suspected uterine anomalies*

IMAGING PARAMETERS FOR A STANDARD EXAMINATION IN THIRD TRIMESTER[3]

- *Fetal cardiac activity, fetal number, and presentation* should be documented. Abnormal heart rate and rhythm should be documented. Ultrasound is also used for the confirmation of malpresentations where Leopold maneuvers may not be sensitive enough. Obstetric management would change with the diagnosis of a malpresentation at term. Multiple gestations require the documentation of additional information: chorionicity, amnionicity, fetal discordancy in growth or CRL and amniotic fluid assessment in each sac by a single vertical pocket.
- A semiquantitative estimate of *amniotic fluid volume (AFV)* should be documented. Either of the parameters can be used such as amniotic fluid index (AFI), single deepest pocket (SDP/MVP), and 2-diameter pocket. For AFI, measure DVP in the 4 quadrants of the uterus that is at least 1 cm wide and is free of fetal parts and cord, while holding the ultrasound transducer perpendicular to the table and parallel to the long axis of the patient's body and add the measurements.
- For oligohydramnios, a cut off value of SVP <2 cm is a preferred criteria over AFI <5 cm since it results in fewer interventions without a significant difference in perinatal outcome. Whereas for polyhydramnios, a cut off of SVP >8 cm or AFI >24 cm can be used. It is preferrable to assess polyhydramnios using AFI.
- For twins single pocket estimation MVP (normal range 2–8 cm) is used.
- The *placental location*, appearance and distance from internal os should be documented. The umbilical cord should be evaluated for number of vessels in the cord and *placental cord insertion site. These should be documented. Also look for placental pathology such as* morbidly adherent placenta and vasa previa using colour Doppler.
- *Fetal weight estimation* can be done from measurements, i.e., BPD, HC, AC and femoral diaphysis length. Scans to assess interval growth velocity should be ideally performed at least 3 weeks apart. A shorter scan interval may result in confusion as even the best weight prediction methods can yield errors as high as +15%. The biometry parameters are plotted against standardized growth charts (e.g., Hadlock, WHO, Intergrowth 21) to assess growth trends.
- *Assessment of fetal wellbeing* in the third trimester includes biophysical profile and additional Doppler parameters, such as umbilical artery Doppler, middle cerebral artery (MCA), ductus venosus and uterine artery Doppler velocimetry.

- *Pregnancy dating* should not be performed in third trimester due to inherent inaccuracy. However if there are no prior antenatal sonography and the patient report late to the clinician, then the head circumference plus femur length can be used as a third trimester dating parameter with a variation of +15 days.
- *Detection of evolving or missed anomalies:* The third trimester scan should look beyond fetal well-being alone, and look for structural survey as well. The must see planes should be evaluated to rule out any evolving anomaly which presents first time in second half of gestation namely CNS abnormalities, genitourinary/GI tract anomalies or cardiac evolving anomalies.

Fetal Growth Surveillance

Fetal growth restriction (FGR) is an important cause of perinatal morbidity and mortality. Timely diagnosis in the antenatal period along with intensive fetal surveillance such as color Doppler can improve the perinatal outcome.

Ultrasound based fetal growth assessment is the modality of choice when there is a suspicion of clinical discrepancy in symphysio-fundal height and gestational age or a high risk pregnancy due to obstetric factor or medical diseases which predispose to FGR.[4]

Accurate estimation of gestational age is a prerequisite before labeling a fetus as small/large for gestational age. Dating pregnancies is best done by early ultrasound examination at 8–14 weeks (CRL <84 mm) or based on HC (if CRL >84 mm). Dating of pregnancy once defined should not be modified as per the subsequent scans.[5]

As per the ISUOG guidelines, EFW may be used to monitor fetal size and growth. For accurately determining interval growth or identifying a growth lag, a preferable time interval between two ultrasound scans of atleast 3 weeks is suggested. However this interval can be shortened when indicated clinically.5

- *AGA* (appropriate-for-gestational age) fetus is one whose size is within the normal range for its gestational age. AGA fetuses typically have individual biometric parameters and/or EFW between the 10th and 90th percentiles **(Fig. 1)**.
- *SGA* (small-for-gestational age) is a fetus whose size is below the cut off threshold for its gestational age. SGA fetuses typically have EFW or AC below the 10th percentile, although 5th centile, 3rd centile, –2SD and Z-score deviation have also been used as cut-offs in the literature **(Fig. 2)**.
- *FGR* (fetal growth restriction) fetus is one that has not achieved its growth potential. Depending upon the period of onset, fetal growth restriction has been classified into early-onset (detected before 32 weeks' gestation) and late-onset (detected after 32 weeks' gestation) types **(Figs. 3A and B)**.

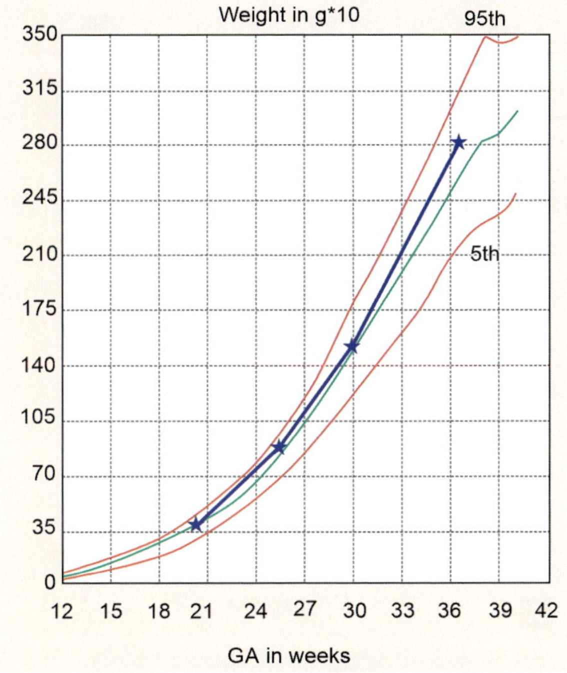

Fig. 1: Appropriate-for-gestational age fetus growth charts.

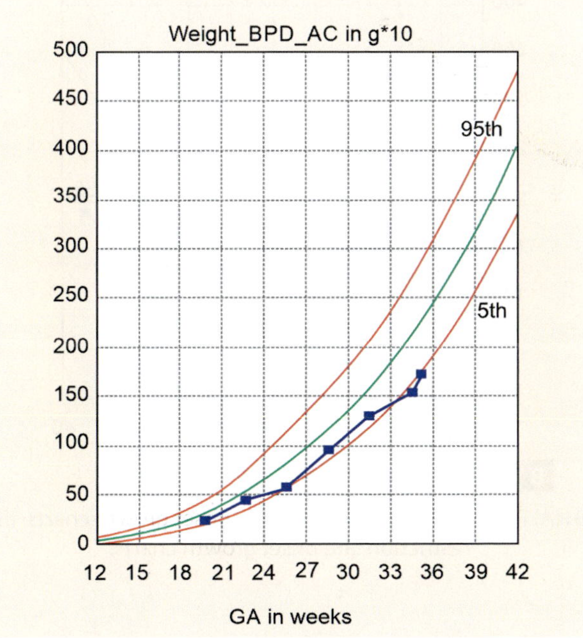

Fig. 2: Small-for-gestational age fetus growth charts.

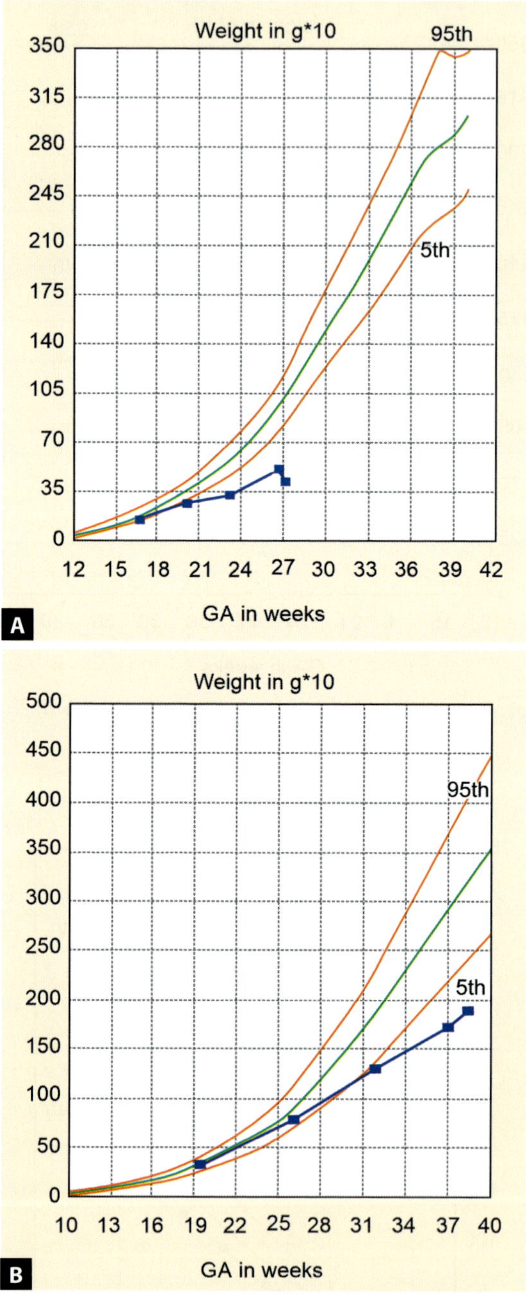

Figs. 3A and B: (A) Fetal growth restriction early onset growth charts; (B) Fetal growth restriction late onset growth charts.

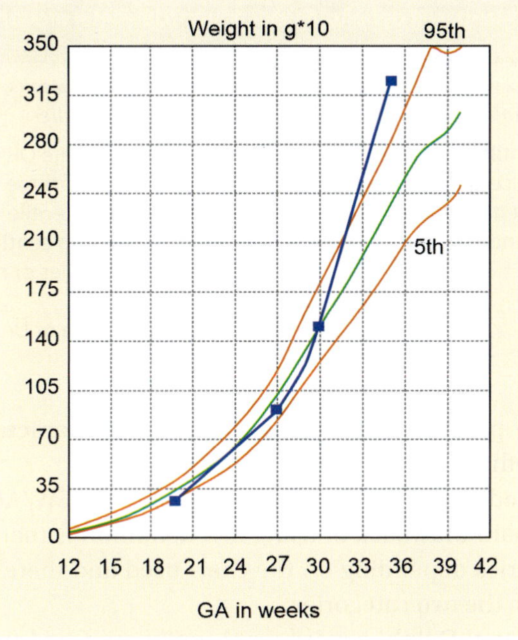

Fig. 4: Large-for-gestational age growth charts.

Another traditional method of classification involves the symmetry of fetal body proportions being indicative of the underlying etiology for FGR. The ISUOG recommendations state that the terms 'symmetrical' and 'asymmetrical' FGR should be abandoned since they do not provide additional information with regard to etiology or prognosis.[5]

- *LGA* (large-for-gestational age) fetus where the fetal size is above cut off threshold for gestational age. LGA typically is defined as EFW or AC above the 90th percentile. Macrosomia at term usually refers to a weight above a fixed cut-off (4,000 or 4,500 g) **(Fig. 4)**. The rationale of identifying macrosomia is to prevent or be prepared for shoulder dystocia which a commonly associated complication. Screening for LGA in the general population may be more accurate when the examination is performed at 36 rather than 32 weeks.

Fetal growth curves have been developed in an attempt to improve the detection rate of SGA, e.g., the Eunice Kennedy Shriver National Institute of Child Health and Human Development (NICHD) Fetal Growth Studies, INTERGROWTH-21st and World Health Organization Multicentre Growth Reference Study (WHO Fetal). The latter two studies on fetal growth started with the assumption that infants and children of well-off parents represent optimal growth in size and that there would be no differences internationally in fetal growth when conditions were optimal.[6-9] Customized growth charts

TABLE 1: Consensus-based definitions for early and late fetal growth restriction (FGR) in absence of congenital anomalies.[5,10]

Early FGR: GA <32 weeks, in absence of congenital anomalies	***Late FGR: GA ≥32 weeks, in absence of congenital anomalies***
AC/EFW <3rd centile or UA-AEDF OR • AC/EFW <10th centile combined with • UtA-PI >95th centile and/or • UA-PI >95th centile	AC/EFW <3rd centile OR At least two out of three of the following: • AC/EFW <10th centile • AC/EFW crossing centiles >2 quartiles on growth centiles or more than 50 centiles • CPR <5th centile or UA-PI >95th centile

have also been proposed according to maternal characteristics (height, weight, parity, ethnicity) and fetal gender.[6-9]

FGR is defined as growth below a cut-off value of EFW/AC < 10th centile. However, the main drawback of using this definition is that the10th centile cut-off value varies depending on the chart used and there is considerable overlap between the two categories.

An international Delphi consensus recently proposed that either of two criteria can be used

EFW/AC below 3rd centile as a sole diagnostic criteria Or EFW/AC below 10th centile PLUS associated criteria (as below). A declining trend in centile or Z score on growth charts warrants additional monitoring **(Table 1)**. ISUOG guidelines recommend the diagnostic criteria for sFGR may be based on Delphi consensus criteria.[5,10]

A diagnosis of FGR should trigger referral to an appropriate unit for individualized management. This will include assessment of fetal well-being in order to identify those fetuses requiring delivery. Antenatal testing modalities include: cardiotocography (non-stress test); basic ultrasound tools such as amniotic fluid index assessment; or advanced modality such as biophysical profile (BPP) score; Color Doppler indices of the umbilical artery, middle cerebral artery or a combination of the two (cerebro-placental ratio); and assessment of ductus venosus flow. Stage based approach to management of FGR has been proposed by Gratacos **(Table 2)**.[11]

Doppler for Diagnosis, Etiology and Surveillance in FGR

Once ultrasound biometry identifies a fetus as SGA (EFW <10th centile), Doppler velocimetry is extremely useful for making the critical differentiation between constitutionally small healthy (<10th centile) fetuses and the pathological growth restricted fetuses and stratify small fetuses which require more surveillance. Doppler flow provides insight into the etiology of fetal growth restriction and is used in monitoring of FGR.

TABLE 2: Stage-based classification and management of FGR.

Stage	*Pathophysiological correlate*	*Criteria (any of)*	*Monitoring*	*GA/mode of delivery*
I	Severe smallness or mild placental insufficiency	• EFW <3rd centile • CPR <p5 • UA PI >p95 • MCA PI <p5 • UtA PI >p95	Weekly	37 weeks LI
II	Severe placental insufficiency	UA AEDV	Biweekly	34 weeks CS
III	Low-suspicion fetal acidosis	• UA REDV • DV-PI >p95	1 – 2 days	30 weeks CS
IV	High-suspicion fetal acidosis	• DV reverse a flow • c CTG <3 ms • FHR decelerations	12 h	26 weeks CS

Umbilical Artery Doppler

American college of Obstetrics and Gynecology recommends use of Umbilical Artery Doppler (UAD) as a standard method for antepartum fetal surveillance in FGR fetus. Its use in SGA fetus is associated with significant reduction in perinatal mortality rates (29% reduction) as well as reduced iatrogenic intervention.[11]

Whereas uterine artery reflects trophoblastic invasion and placental development, Umbilical Artery Doppler reflects placental function and indicates degree of placental insufficiency. It correlates with the tertiary villous architecture and blood flow resistance. Umbilical artery Doppler resistance is elevated if at least 30% of fetal villous vasculature becomes abnormal. Umbilical Artery absent diastolic flow indicates 60–70% damage to villous vascular architecture and an increased risk of perinatal mortality **(Figs. 5A to D)**.

Measurements of umbilical artery Doppler indices should be made in a free cord loop. Impedance is highest at the fetal end and lowest at placental end. S/D, RI, PI reference value varies at different gestational age and they can be plotted on centile charts. The PI offers the advantage of smallest measured error, narrower reference limit and advantage of ongoing numeric analysis even when diastolic flow is absent or reversed.[12]

Middle Cerebral Artery Doppler Flow

Middle Cerebral Artery Doppler (MCA) flows depict fetal response to hypoxemia. The fetus adapts itself to chronic hypoxemia with preferentially diverting blood to vital organs (brain, heart and adrenals) leading to increased diastolic flow in the MCA and decrease in doppler indices (Brain sparing effect/Cerebral vasodilatation/Centralization). MCA is particularly valuable

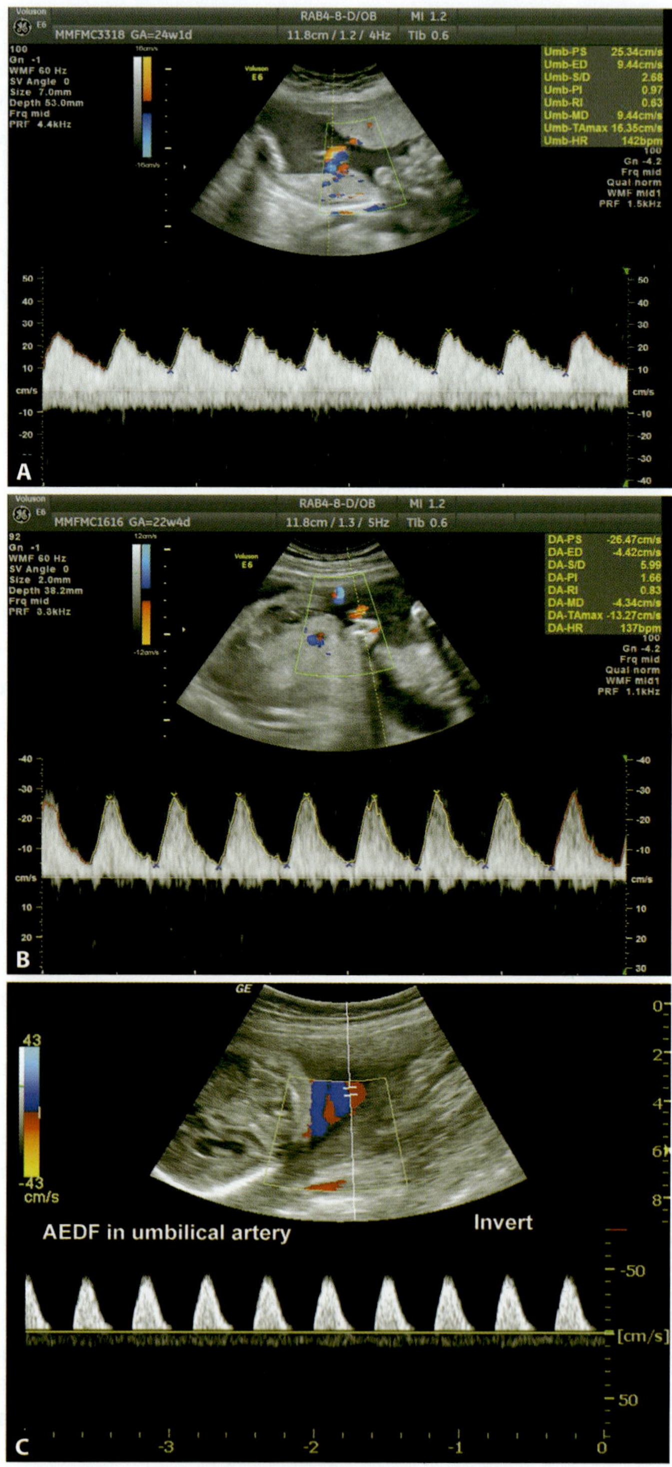

RAB4-8-D/OB
MI 1.2
MMFMC3318 GA=24w1d
11.8cm / 1.2 / 4Hz
Tib 0.6
Umb-PS 25.34cm/s
Umb-ED 9.44cm/s
Umb-S/D 2.68
Umb-PI 0.97
Umb-RI 0.63
Umb-MD 9.44cm/s
Umb-TAmax 16.35cm/s
Umb-HR 142bpm
A
RAB4-8-D/OB
MI 1.2
MMFMC1616 GA=22w4d
11.8cm / 1.3 / 5Hz
Tib 0.6
DA-PS -26.47cm/s
DA-ED -4.42cm/s
DA-S/D 5.99
DA-PI 1.66
DA-RI 0.83
DA-MD -4.34cm/s
DA-TAmax -13.27cm/s
DA-HR 137bpm
B
43
-43
cm/s
AEDF in umbilical artery
Invert
-50
[cm/s]
50
C

Figs. 5A to C

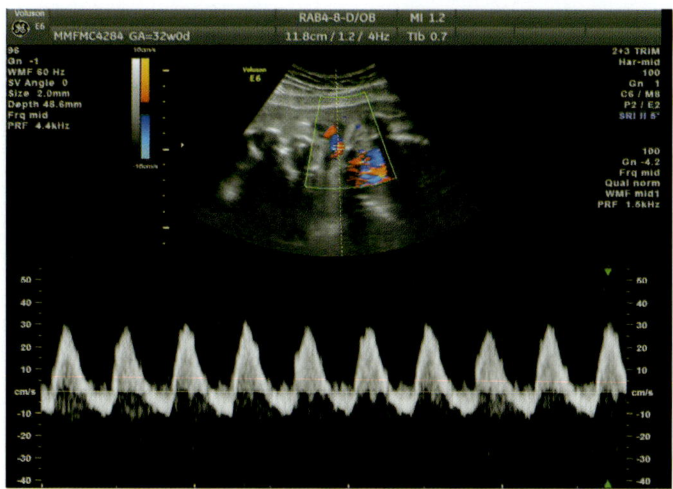

Fig. 5D

Figs. 5A to D: (A) Normal umbilical artery Doppler; (B) High resistance umbilical artery Doppler; (C) Absent diastolic flow umbilical artery Doppler; (D) Reversed diastolic flow umbilical artery Doppler.

for the identification and prediction of adverse outcome among late-onset FGR, independently of the UA Doppler, which is often normal in these fetuses **(Figs. 6A and B)**.[11]

While evaluating MCA for pulse wave doppler measurement, sample gate should be placed at proximal third of the MCA, near the origin in the internal carotid artery. Systolic velocity is inversely variable with distance from origin point.

The highest point of the waveform is considered as PSV (Peak systolic velocity in cm/s). Fetal middle cerebral artery doppler for peak systolic velocity is a non-invasive means to assess fetal anemia in Rh isoimmunized pregnancies.[12]

Cerebroplacental ratio: Cerebroplacental ratio (CPR) is the ratio between the middle cerebral artery pulsatility index (MCA-PI) and the umbilical artery pulsatility index (UA-PI). The CPR is essentially a diagnostic index that improves the sensitivity of UA and MCA alone in late onset FGR. A reduced MCA PI or MCA/umbilical artery PI ratio (cerebroplacental ratio <1) are early signs of hypoxemia in late FGR.

Ductus venosus doppler: DV is the strongest marker among all Doppler parameters to predict the short-term risk of fetal death in early-onset FGR. DV flow waveforms become altered only in advanced stages of fetal compromise Thus, absent or reversed 'a' wave pattern is normally considered sufficient to recommend delivery at any gestational age, after completion of steroids **(Figs. 7A and B)**.[11]

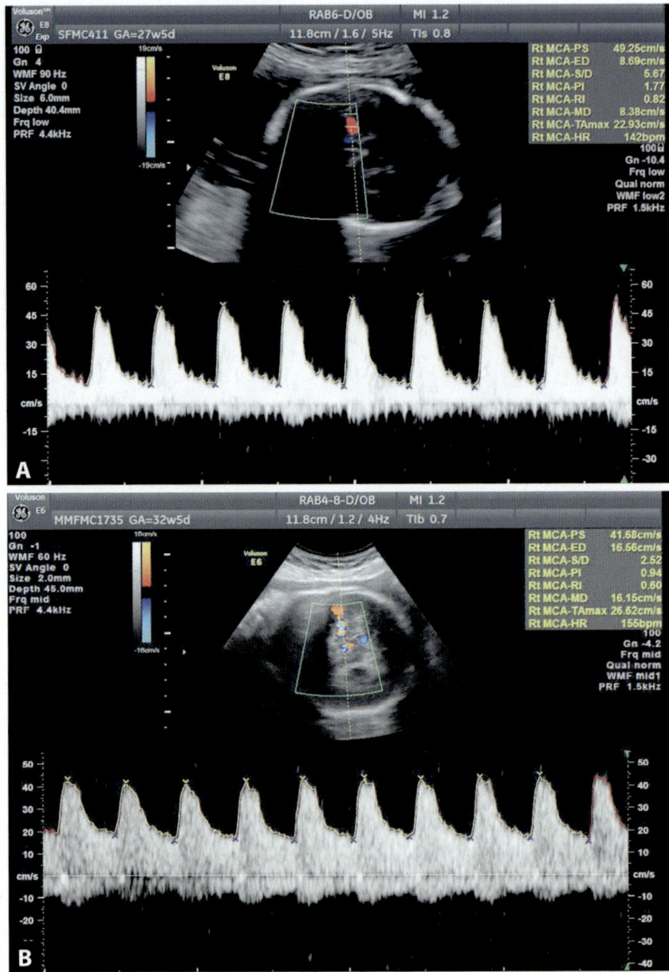

Figs. 6A and B: (A) Middle cerebral artery normal Doppler; (B) Middle cerebral artery Doppler showing brain sparing effect.

The waveform is usually triphasic, (M-shape) that reflects pressure volume changes in right atria through cardiac cycle. Normal blood flow in DV is forward flow throughout the cardiac cycle. Doppler measurement is best achieved in the sagittal plane from the anterior lower fetal abdomen.[12]

Based upon Doppler changes, Stage based approach to management of FGR has been proposed by Gratacos **(Table 2)**.[11]

Antepartum Fetal Surveillance

Biophysical Profile

Fetal biophysical scoring originally described by Manning et al, is based on assessment of five discrete biophysical variables. Four of the

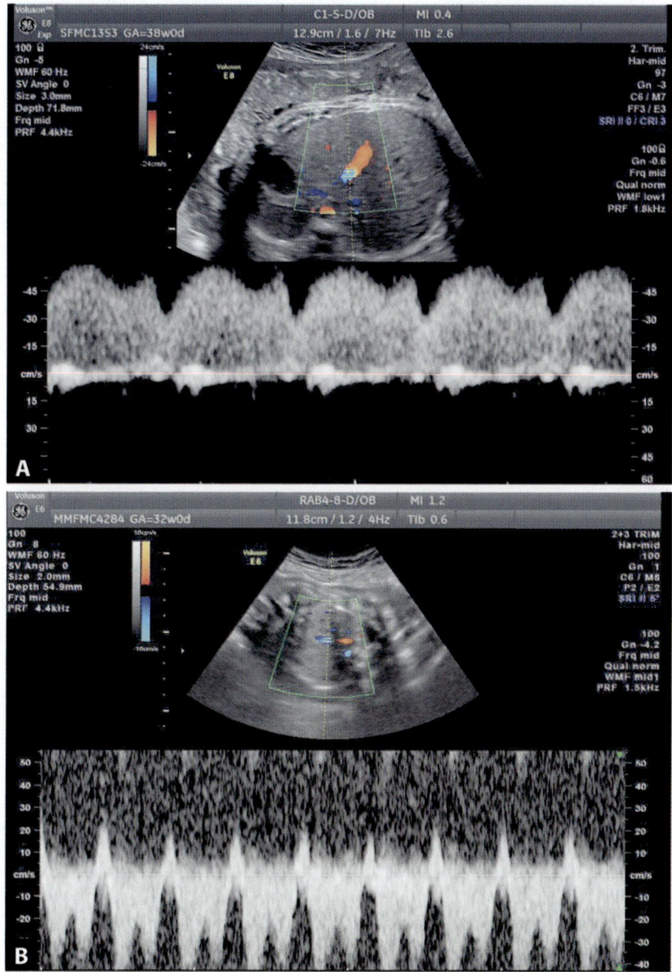

Figs. 7A and B: (A) Ductus venosus normal Doppler; (B) Reversed a wave in ductus venosus Doppler.

variables (except NST) namely, fetal breathing movements, gross body movements, fetal tone, and amniotic volume (fetal urine output) are monitored simultaneously by dynamic ultrasound imaging. These variables are dependent on the integrity of the fetal CNS and show abnormal response in a compromised fetus **(Table 3)**.[13]

A composite value of 8 or 10 indicates that the fetal status is reassuring or normal as long as the score of 8 does not include an abnormal amniotic fluid volume. The presence of oligohydramnios demands further testing or delivery, irrespective of the composite score value. A score of 6 is equivocal and requires further testing in 24 hours if less than 37 weeks or consideration for delivery if >37 weeks. A BPP score of 4 or less is suggestive of fetal compromise and an indication for delivery if salvageable weeks of gestation. If gestational

TABLE 3: Manning's biophysical profile scoring.[13]

Variable	*Score 2*	*Score 0*
Fetal Breathing movements	≥30 seconds of sustained fetal breathing movements in 30 minutes	<30 seconds of fetal breathing movements in 30 minutes
Fetal movements	≥3 gross body movements in 30 minutes. Simultaneous limb and trunk movements are considered as single movement	≤2 gross body movements in 30 minutes
Fetal tone	At least one episode of motion of a limb from a position of flexion to extension and return to flexion	Fetus in a position of semi- or full- limb extension with no return to flexion with movement; absence of fetal movement is counted as absent tone
Fetal reactivity	Two or more FHR accelerations of at least 15 beats/minute and lasting at least 15 seconds and associated with fetal movements in 40 minutes	No acceleration or less than 2 accelerations of FHR in 40 minutes
Quantitative amniotic fluid volume	SVP ≥2 cm	SVP <2 cm
Maximal score	10	
Minimal score		0

age less than 32 weeks then extended monitoring during the time of maternal steroid administration maybe appropriate and individualized.[14]

The false negative rate of BPP is 0.7/1000, a value better than that of the NST i.e. antepartum death of a structurally normal fetus within one week of a normal BPP. The negative predictive value of BPP is similar to NST (98.5%). The positive predictive value of an abnormal test is 50.8%. More than 97% of the pregnancies tested have normal test results.[14]

The gradual hypoxia concept suggest that not all variables carry same power. Fetal heart rate reactivity (NST), amniotic fluid volume and fetal breathing movements are the most powerful markers of perinatal outcome. Amniotic fluid volume reflects chronic changes in intrauterine oxygenation, whereas the other 4 variables are indicators of a more acute state.[14]

Biophysical profile is time consuming and requires ultrasound training. However, it has no contraindications and involves no risk for the mother or the fetus. It is both more sensitive and more specific in predicting abnormal outcome than the NST.

Modified Biophysical Profile

Several abbreviated modifications of the original BPP have been introduced in order to rationalize the use of human and equipment resources without impairing test performance.

The modified BPP, proposed by Vintzileos et al, describes a testing scheme using the most powerful components of the BPP, NST (using Acoustic stimulation test, AST) with an evaluation of the amniotic fluid. Thus, this modification assesses both the most sensitive acute marker (fetal heart rate tracing) and chronic marker (amniotic fluid volume) of fetal well-being.[15] AST is used to shorten the time required to achieve a reactive NST.

The test has excellent negative and positive predictive values. It is easy to interpret, has clearly defined end points, and can be performed in a short period of time about 20 minutes[15]:

- If both NST and amniotic fluid index are normal, weekly fetal surveillance with MBPP is continued.
- If both tests are abnormal (Nonreactive NST, decreased amniotic fluid volume) and the gestational age is beyond 36 weeks the preferred option would be delivery. If gestational age is below 36 weeks, then management is individualized. Doppler studies, full BPP, or delivery may be used to depending on the circumstances.
- If amniotic fluid volume is decreased but the NST is reactive, a search for indicators of placental insufficiency or undiagnosed rupture of membranes need to be undertaken and management will be dependent on the final diagnosis.
- If amniotic fluid is normal and NST is Nonreactive, further testing with full BPP or Doppler is indicated.

Overall, the MBPP has a false positive rate (60 %) comparable to the NST, but higher than a full BPP. The false negative rate (0.8/1,000), decreased testing time and the ease of performance of MBPP make it an excellent approach for the evaluation of high-risk patients in large numbers. The ACOG [American College of Obstetricians & Gynecologists] guidelines in 2014, have concluded that the modified BPP test is as predictive of fetal well-being as other approaches to biophysical fetal surveillance[15].

Amniotic Fluid Volume (AFV)

The American College of Obstetricians and Gynecologists ACOG has defined Oligohydramnios as SVP <2 cm or AFI <5 cm. For oligohydramnios look for additional USG parameters including Fetal growth and color doppler, KUB system for evaluation for Bilateral renal agenesis, renal disorders or obstructive lesions and target history for premature rupture of membranes.

If polyhydramnios is seen, rule out common associations like maternal diabetes, fetal abnormalities (mostly gastrointestinal obstructions causing swallowing impairment like cleft lip, neck tumors, esophageal and duodenal atresia, cardiac and CNS anomalies), chromosomal and genetic abnormalities, conditions that result in anemia and hyperdynamic circulation like placental tumors and fetal infections and idiopathic in 50–60% of cases.

Detection of Late Evolving Fetal Anomalies

A 3rd trimester structural survey is important to screen for evolving anomalies as they may manifest for the first time in later gestation. 50% of all anomalies are detected prior to 24 weeks and other half remain undiagnosed or detected after 24 weeks. Often the early detection of anomaly maybe missed due to smaller size of organs (at earlier stage of development) precluding the assessment, unfavorable fetal position or poor ultrasound machine resolution.

Some anomalies which manifest as functional impairment (e.g. urogenital) are detected for the first time in the third trimester.[16] Also the phenotypic expression of some abnormalities become apparent only at a later gestation, such as short limbs in the case of achondroplasia, dilated bowel in the case of bowel atresia or abnormal shape of the head in the case of craniosynostosis. Some of the abnormalities develops only during the third trimester, such as ovarian cysts in response to maternal estrogenic stimulation or ventriculomegaly following fetal brain hemorrhage or maternal infection.

These anomalies might be overlooked if the third trimester sonography is not done in view to detect anomalies. Among the various anomalies detected in the third trimester about 50% are comprised of central nervous system and the urogenital system. Other organ systems that commonly manifest late anomalies are musculoskeletal and gastrointestinal system.[16]

The potential benefits of diagnosing a fetal anomaly in third trimester, previously undiagnosed, include planning the location, timing, and route of delivery. It may be modified in order to improve perinatal care, the opportunity to arrange for in-utero transfer to an appropriate level of neonatal care; allow the parents time and counseling to prepare for the birth of an anomalous child; perform prenatal genetic analysis such as third-trimester amniocentesis and plan neonatal counseling and follow-up.

In special circumstances where grave consequences are expected for the child then, as per legal permissions (national guidelines) , termination of pregnancy along with feticide, may be opted.

The must see planes along with common conditions to rule out are listed as below **(Table 4)**.

Fetal CNS Abnormalities

About 15% of pregnancies with a fetal CNS abnormality first detected in the third trimester have a previous normal second-trimester anomaly scan.

TABLE 4: USG planes in third trimester and abnormal findings pointing to potential fetal conditions.

Plane (ultrasound)	*Abnormal findings to watch for*	*Late appearing Potential conditions to rule out*
Head biometry BPD and HC plane	Below -3SD usually associated with cortical anomalies and a sloping forehead	Microcephaly
Head BPD plane—cerebral cortex	Sulcation and gyration	• Poorly formed sulci gyri—lissencephaly • Excessive sulci gyri — polymicrogyria • *Note:* Cerebral cortical defect are difficult to diagnose on USG and may require MRI
Head axial planes—ventricles plane and cerebellar plane	• *Symmetry of the hemisphere* • *Ventricular plane:* Lateral Ventricle measurement >10 mm • Thalamic plane • Cerebellar plane	• Ventriculomegaly • Posterior fossa anomaly • Vein of Galen aneurysm • Arachnoid cyst
Heart	• Situs, size and symmetry of the heart • 4 chamber view, outflow tracts • 3 Vessel Trachea view • Watch for Caliber of great vessels, forward flow, stenosis or regurgitation of flow, chamber asymmetry	• Rhabdomyoma • Great vessels—pulmonary atresia or stenosis, coarctation aorta
Chest	• Sagittal and coronal view and assessment of diaphragm • Any masses—size, midline shift , LHR ratio for CDH • For pleural effusion: Volume of fluid collection and lung volume , hydrops if any	• Congenital diaphragmatic hernia • Pleural effusion • Congenital pulmonary airway malformation
Abdomen	• Any dilated bowel loop • Small bowel -8 mm and large bowel 18 mm • For echogenic bowel, reduce gain setting and check if foci are as echogenic as bone • Associated finding of FGR or TORCH stigma, liver calcification • If any atresia then proximal segment distention • More higher lesions will present with polyhydramnios	• Abdominal Cysts and echogenic bowel • Duodenal atresia • Small and large bowel atresia or Volvulus • ascites

Contd...

Contd...

Plane (ultrasound)	*Abnormal findings to watch for*	*Late appearing Potential conditions to rule out*
KUB	Abdominal coronal plane to check if: • Kidneys bilaterally present, bladder • Confirm renal artery arising from aorta • Check renal parenchyma—rule out echogenic or cortex thinning, loss of architecture, cysts if any • If hydronephrosis is seen then measure renal pelvis in axial plane • Renal pelvis anteroposterior (AP) diameter cutoff value in the third trimester is >7 mm, and an AP diameter >15 mm is associated with an increased risk for need of postnatal surgery	• Hydronephrosis • MCDK • PCKD

The most common central nervous system anomalies detected late is mild ventriculomegaly.

Two groups of brain abnormalities that can be diagnosed only in the third trimester are developmental anomalies and acquired lesions. Acquired lesions, include as stroke, hemorrhage, infection and tumors, and the former group includes developmental anomalies such as Vein of Galen malformation, and malformations of cortical development which include microcephaly, megalencephaly, lissencephaly/subcortical band heterotopia spectrum, cobblestone complex, heterotopia, polymicrogyria and schizencephaly which become evident during rapid brain enlargement after the end of the proliferation and migration period (2–5 months of gestation).

Abnormalities of sulci-gyri may be due to single gene disorders or other genetic causes, hence the importance of detailed history cannot be over-emphasized.

Fetal Genitourinary Anomalies

Hydronephrosis is the most common genitourinary abnormality diagnosed at the third trimester scan.

Renal abnormalities include urinary tract dilatation disorders like pelvi-ureteric junction obstruction, vesico-ureteric reflux or obstruction, partial obstructive posterior urethral valves present with varying grades of hydronephrosis with/without hydroureter and/or oligohydramnios at different gestational age depending upon the severity of obstruction and level of obstruction. All urinary tract dilatation require 3–4 weekly antenatal monitoring for worsening, oligohydramnios, cortical thickness and echogenicity and fetal maturity so as to decide time of delivery balancing the risk of prematurity versus worsening renal function.

Fetal Gastrointestinal Anomalies

Higher the obstruction earlier is the time of presentation in antenatal period by visualization of polyhydramnios and dilated bowel loops proximal to the obstruction while lower bowel obstruction in the colon or rectum may not become obvious even in the late gestation as the fluid is resorbed in the upstream small bowel and colonic loops.

Prenatal diagnosis of bowel obstruction and referral to tertiary center with early neonatal surgical correction reduces morbidity due to aspiration pneumonia or further abdominal distention with respiratory embarrassment if undiagnosed.

Congenital Lung Malformations

Congenital Pulmonary Adenomatoid Malformation (CPAM) and broncho-pulmonary sequestration (BPS) are fetal lung masses where the natural history may be progression/regression or remains stable antenatally and hence require monitoring in the third trimester for worsening or development of hydrops. Congenital Pulmonary Airway Malformation Volume Ratio (CVR) helps determine the risk of development of hydrops and is an important parameter which is to be considered when counseling such patients. A CVR of ≤1.6 at presentation suggests that the risk of hydrops developing is low in the absence of a dominant large cyst.

Congenital diaphragmatic hernia is a malformation with important implications due to high mortality. If diagnosed before 26 weeks gestation with associated liver herniation and a low lung to head circumference ratio (LHR <1) they have a relatively poor prognosis with conventional therapy after birth. The mainstay of management includes meticulous initial evaluation of LHR and extent of liver herniation, chromosomal analysis, antenatal monitoring of the fetus for signs of worsening, cardiac dysfunction and development of hydrops in the third trimester, delivery near term at a tertiary care center with NICU set-up, standard protocols for management of neonate at birth including initial intubation, stabilization and surgical management.

Cardiac Anomalies

Perinatal morbidity and mortality improves drastically when cardiac anomalies are diagnosed prenatally as it gives opportunity of optimum management in a tertiary care unit. Relatively non-lethal with good post-surgical results include isolated ventricular septal defects, isolated transposition of great vessels, Fallot's tetralogy with good size pulmonary artery, total anomalous pulmonary venous connections and milder varieties of coarctation of aorta may manifest at later gestation. Also rare conditions like cardiac soft tissue tumors like rhabdomyoma are almost always detected in the late trimester.

Further antenatal monitoring is necessary in the late gestation by an expert fetal medicine/fetal cardiac specialized center for worsening of cardiac function, signs of heart failure or development of hydrops and deciding the timing/mode of delivery at a center with good neonatal intensive care unit for initial assessment and stabilization.

Fetal Musculoskeletal Abnormalities

Diseases of the musculoskeletal system like achondroplasia though rare manifest in the third trimester after 26 weeks. Although these are non-lethal skeletal dysplasia without mental impairment, it is nevertheless of great importance to prepare the parents and to inform them prenatally.

As per a recent study on 52,400 study population on the value of routine ultrasound at 35–37 weeks of gestation in the diagnosis of fetal abnormalities, the incidence of fetal abnormality was 1.9% and 24.8% were detected for the first time at 35–37 weeks.[16] Prenatal diagnosis even if diagnosed late in gestation may have a significant impact on the perinatal management of the fetus with a surgically correctable congenital anomaly. A routine ultrasound during the third trimester is therefore justified.

ROLE OF THIRD TRIMESTER ULTRASOUND IN PLACENTAL LOCALIZATION AND ACCRETA SPECTRUM

Placental location and its relationship with the internal cervical os should be assessed in the third trimester scan. This is specially indicated when a low lying placenta or placenta previa is diagnosed in the mid-trimester scan or when there is a painless episode of bleeding. The distance of the edge of the placenta from the internal os and the position of cord insertion should be assessed. Placenta previa is a risk factor for abnormal cord insertion such as velamentous cord insertion and vasa previa and these anomalies should be ruled out when assessing women with suspected placenta previa in the third trimester. If the placenta is low, subsequent scans are performed as indicated, to assess whether the placenta has moved away from the internal os. Transvaginal ultrasound is preferred for accurate localization of the placental site, particularly when the transabdominal approach is difficult in maternal obesity, uterine scar or fibroids or a posteriorly placed behind the fetal head. If the leading placental edge is more than 20 mm from the internal os, vaginal birth is considered a safe option.

Women with major placenta previa or a uterine scar may be offered a scan at around 28 weeks to rule out placenta accreta and plan mode of delivery, while women with minor placenta previa may be assessed later in the third trimester.

Placenta Accreta Spectrum

Morbidly adherent placenta (PAS) can occur when placenta is low lying along with a prior Cesarean birth or uterine surgery, including myomectomy or multiple curettages. Hence a third trimester scan should document the position of placenta (anterior or posterior) and its relation to the cervix and scar area and for indicators of placenta accreta.

It is better to error on the side of caution and consider every woman with placenta previa and a prior Cesarean birth or uterine surgery as a potential case of PAS. A prenatally diagnosed PAS is associated with less hemorrhagic complication and should be managed by a well equipped center with multidisciplinary team and surgical expertise of morbidly adherent placenta.

Standardized descriptors of PAS have been described which have a diagnostic accuracy of almost 90% (17). They include:

- Loss of the retroplacental clear zone **(Fig. 8A)**
- Myometrial thinning,
- Interruption of bladder wall interface
- Presence of a placental bulge
- Focal exophytic mass
- Uterovesical hypervascularity
- Placental lacunae and
- Bridging vessels **(Fig. 8B)**

Vasa previa is diagnosed by using transvaginal ultrasound and with color Doppler demonstration of the umbilical cord inserting into membranes over the cervix, from where unprotected vessels run into the placenta. Transvaginal ultrasound with color Doppler is a useful tool for screening vasa previa in cases of second-trimester low-lying placenta, bilobed placenta or placenta with succenturiate lobes, and multiple gestation in the third trimester.

GESTATIONAL AGE FOR THIRD TRIMESTER ULTRASOUND

The timing of the third-trimester scan, varies between 28 to 32 and 36 weeks. It should be individualized based on maternal and fetal risk factors and local objectives and resources. The anatomical examination is technically easier at 28–32 weeks. On the other hand, any growth deviations (SGA/LGA) is best detected towards 36 weeks in low-risk pregnancies. In pregnancies at higher risk of complications, it is advisable to do ultrasound examination at 28 to 32 weeks or earlier (18).

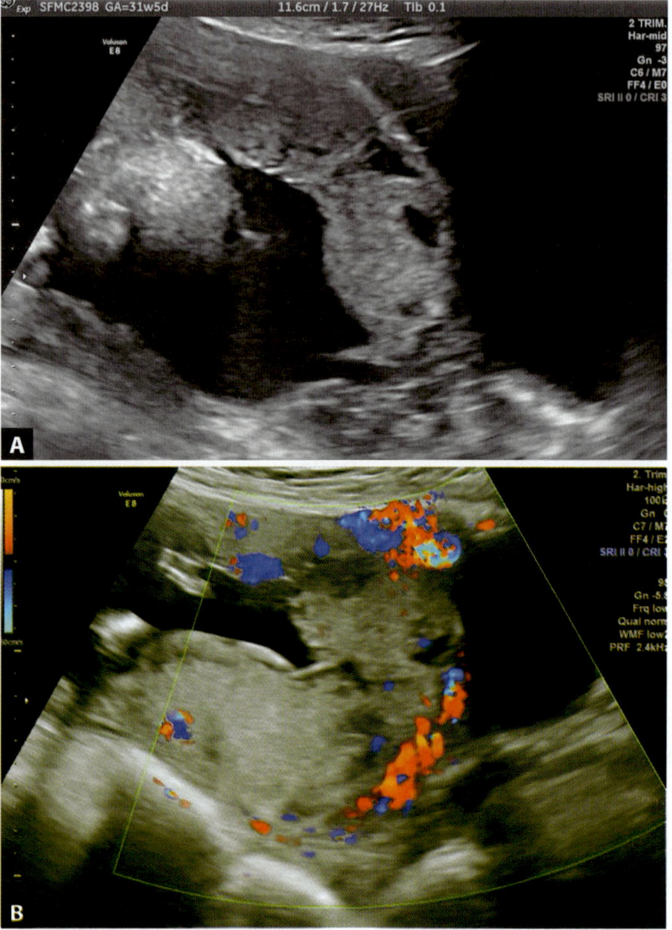

Figs. 8A and B: (A) Placenta accreta loss of retroplacental clear zone; (B) Placenta accreta with bridging vessels.

INTRAPARTUM USG

The use of ultrasound has been proposed to aid in the management of labor. Traditionally, the assessment and management of a woman in labor is based upon clinical findings, However, clinical examination of head station and position is inaccurate and subjective, especially when caput succedaneum impairs palpation of the sutures and fontanels.

Several studies have demonstrated that ultrasound examination is more accurate and reproducible than clinical examination in the diagnosis of fetal head position and station and in the prediction of arrest of labor. At present till there is a consensus on when and which parameters to use, ultrasound in labor should be used as an adjunct and not a substitute for clinical examination. Ultrasound in labor can be performed using a transabdominal approach, mainly to determine head and spine position, or a transperineal approach, for assessment of head station and position at low stations.[19]

When to use:

- Tardy progress or arrest in second stage of labor
- Assess the descent/station of the head prior to instrumental assisted vaginal delivery. Combination of Ultrasound assessment and digital examination prior to instrumental vaginal delivery is more accurate compared with digital examination alone in the diagnosis of fetal head position.
- Head malpresentation suspected

Parameters to assess:

- *Fetal head and spine position:* Sonographic assessment of fetal head position is best performed by transabdominal imaging in axial and sagittal planes. Placing the ultrasound probe transversely at the level of maternal suprapubic region, visualize the fetal head.

  Position can be described by depicting a circle in a clock: positions ≥02.30 and ≤03.30 is left occiput transverse (LOT); positions ≥08.30 and ≤ 09.30 as right occiput transverse (ROT); positions >03.30 and <08.30 is recorded as occiput posterior; and positions >09.30 and <02.30 as occiput anterior.
- *Fetal head station and descent* is assessed by transperineal ultrasound in the midsaggital plane with the probe placed between the two labia majora.

  Angle of progression: The AoP is the angle between the long axis of the pubic bone and a line from the lowest edge of the pubis drawn tangential to the deepest bony part of the fetal skull. AoP cut-off value of 120° predicts an easy vacuum delivery.
- *Head attitude and malpresentation:* The longest recognizable axis of the fetal head and the long axis of the pubic symphysis, measured in a midsagittal transperineal view. It is classified as 'head down' (angle <0°), 'horizontal' (angle 0°–30°) and 'head up' (angle >30°).

  Midline angle (MLA): It is measured in the axial plane using a transperineal approach: the echogenic line interposed between the two cerebral hemispheres (midline) is identified, and MLA is the angle between this line and the anteroposterior axis of the maternal pelvis. It utilizes the angle of head rotation as an indicator of birth progress.

CONCLUSION

The third trimester antenatal scan is a highly informative, often underutilized tool. It gives crucial information about fetal wellbeing, growth with color doppler assessment, placental position, liquor estimation, fetal presentation as well as anatomical assessment for evolving anomaly if any. These parameters are decision making for an obstetrician prior to delivery. The timing of delivery, mode of delivery, need of tertiary center or NICU availability or need of in utero transfer can be precisely determined only after the third trimester ultrasound assessment. A handy checklist or knowledge of "what to look for" can be a pivot to influence perinatal and neonatal outcomes. The recently published ISUOG third trimester guidelines define a third trimester ultrasound as a standard of care in antenatal management. This article is focused on harnessing the potential of ultrasound in third trimester and labor in order to improve outcomes.

KEY POINTS

- Five basic parameters to see in third trimester (after documenting FHR):
    1. Presenting part, rule out multiple loops of nuchal cord
    2. Placental position, rule out low lying placenta
    3. Liquor assessment
    4. *Growth assessment:* Estimate fetal weight with biometry parameter BPD HC AC FL
    5. *Cervical length:* If risk of late preterm
- Do an anatomical *survey as a basic screening in every scan.* This will lead to identification of evolving or missed anomalies.
- Keep alert for morbidly adherent placenta in previously scarred uterus with anterior placenta.
- If biometry shows growth lag (below 10th centile), need of color doppler assessment and assigning a stage to FGR (as per Barcelona classification) for monitoring and planning time and mode of delivery.
- For twins use biometry with color Doppler always to rule out selective FGR and discordance in twin. A discordance more than 15-20% affects perinatal outcome.
- Useful tool for near term evaluation of fetal wellbeing is a modified BPP (NST plus AFI) as it combines acute status of fetus (via NST) and chronic status i.e., placental function (via AFI).

REFERENCES

1. Guidelines on use of ultrasonography during pregnancy; Ministry of Health and Family Welfare, Government of India.
2. WHO recommendations on antenatal care for a positive pregnancy experience, 2016: WHO Press, World Health Organization, Geneva, Switzerland.
3. AIUM ACR ACOG SMFM SRU Practice parameters for performance of standard diagnostic ultrasound examination, J Ultrasound Med. 2018;9999:1-12.
4. Ultrasound in pregnancy. Practice Bulletin No. 175. American College of Obstetricians and Gynecologists. Obstet Gynecol. 2016;128:e241-56.

5. ISUOG Practice guidelines: ultrasound assessment of fetal biometry and growth. Ultrasound Obstet Gynecol. 2019;53:715-23.
6. Buck Louis GM, Grewal J, Albert PS, et al. Racial/ethnic standards for fetal growth: the NICHD Fetal Growth Studies. Am J Obstet Gynecol. 2015;213:449. e1-41.
7. Stirnemann J, Villar J, Salomon LJ, et al. International estimated fetal weight standards of the INTERGROWTH-21st Project. Ultrasound Obstet Gynecol. 2017;49:478-86.
8. Kiserud T, Piaggio G, Carroli G, et al. The World Health Organization fetal growth charts: a multinational longitudinal study of ultrasound biometric measurements and estimated fetal weight. PLOS Med. 2017;14:e1002220.
9. Jason Gardosi, Andre Francis et al. Customised growth charts: rationale, validation and clinical results. AJOG. 2018;S609-617.
10. Gordijn SJ Beune IM et al. Consensus definition of fetal growth restriction: a Delphi procedure. Ultrasound Obstet Gynecol. 2016;48:333-9.
11. Francesc Figueras , Eduard Gratacós. Update on the Diagnosis and Classification of Fetal Growth Restriction and Proposal of a Stage-Based Management Protocol. Fetal Diagn Ther. 2014;36:86-98 DOI: 10.1159/000357592
12. ISUOG Practice Guidelines: use of Doppler ultrasonography in obstetrics Ultrasound Obstet Gynecol. 2013;41:233-9.
13. Manning FA, Platt LD, Sipos L: Antepartum fetal evaluation : Development of a fetal biophysical profile score. Am J Obstet Gynecol. 1980;136:787.
14. ACOG Practice Bulletin Number 145: Antepartum Fetal Surveillance. Obstet Gynecol. 2014;124:182-92.
15. Miller DA, Rabello YA, Paul RH: The modified biophysical profile: Antepartum testing in the 1990s. Am J Obstet Gynecol. 1996;174:812.
16. Ficara A, Syngelak . Value of routine ultrasound examination at 35–37 weeks' gestation in diagnosis of fetal abnormalities . Ultrasound Obstet Gynecol 2019. Published online in Wiley Online Library (wileyonlinelibrary.com). DOI: 10.1002/uog.20857
17. Jauniaux E, D'Antonio F, Bhide A, Prefumo F, Silver RM, Hussein AM, Shainker SA, Chantraine F, Alfirevic Z, Delphi consensus expert panel. Modified Delphi study of ultrasound signs associated with placenta accreta spectrum. Ultrasound Obstet Gynecol. 2023;61:518-25.
18. ISUOG Practice Guidelines: performance of third-trimester obstetric ultrasound scan. Ultrasound Obstet Gynecol. 2024;63:131-47.
19. ISUOG Practice Guidelines: intrapartum ultrasound. Ultrasound Obstet Gynecol. 2018;52:128-39. Published online in Wiley Online Library (wileyonlinelibrary. com). DOI: 10.1002/uog.19072 isuog.org GUIDELINES

CHAPTER

Ultrasound in Placental Abnormalities

Chinmayee Ratha

INTRODUCTION

The placenta is a unique organ which develops in pregnancy and is of pivotal importance in fetal viability. Placental dysfunction has been well established as the underlying cause of multiple pregnancy complications like fetal growth restriction or pre-eclampsia; in many other pregnancy related issues the role of the placenta is being unraveled as technology is advancing in prenatal diagnostics. Placental function markers like PAPP-A, PlGF, SFlt among others have found their place in biochemistry-based evaluation of pregnancy complications. The ultrasound assessment of placental structure and hemodynamics has also gained importance in evaluation of pregnancy conditions and thus this chapter is focused on the ultrasound evaluation of the placenta.

PLACENTA IN EARLY PREGNANCY

In early pregnancy ultrasound the placenta development is assessed in its initial stages as an echogenic "decidual reaction" around the developing gestational sac. As evident is **Figure 1**, this decidual reaction is more prominent in the region that will develop into the future placenta.

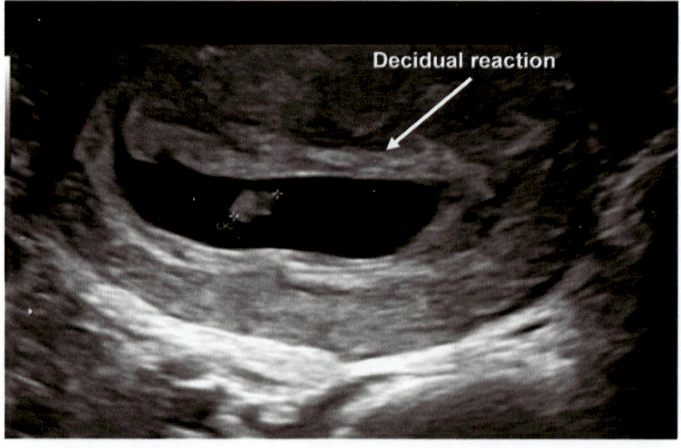

Fig. 1: Decidual reaction in early pregnancy.

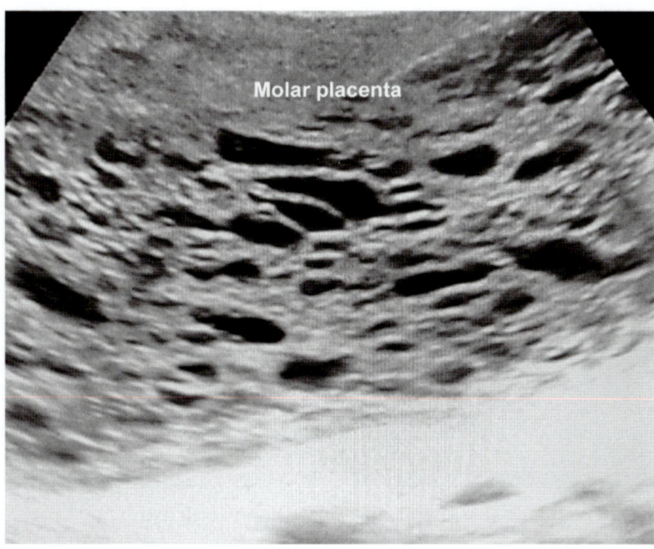

Fig. 2: Molar placenta.

The choriodecidual structure represents the *decidua basalis* in the gestational period of 6–12 weeks and after 12 weeks the development of the chorion frondosum leads to defining of 3 layers in the placenta namely:

- The basal plate
- Placental substance
- The chorionic plate.

The basal plate may not always be perceptible unless calcified. The placental substance has a diffuse granular pattern and the chorionic plate has a strong acoustic surface.[1]

Sometimes the normal placental development is not seen and the uterus is seen filled with cystic spaces which may be representing molar pregnancy **(Fig. 2)**.

A very important aspect of first trimester placental evaluation is in multiple pregnancy to establish chorionicity. When a small "twin peak" sign is seen between two placentae, it can be labelled as dichorionic gestation based on the characteristic "lambda sign" as seen in **Figure 3**.

In case the twin peak sign is missing and the membrane arises directly from the placental surface then we assign monochorionicity based on the "T sign" as shown in **Figure 4**.

PLACENTA IN MIDTRIMESTER

The midtrimester placenta appears as a uniformly echogenic structure along uterine wall, with a deep hypoechoic band separating it from normal uterine myometrium in **Figure 5**. The echogenicity of the normal placenta is typically "intermediate" between echogenicity of bone and viscera.

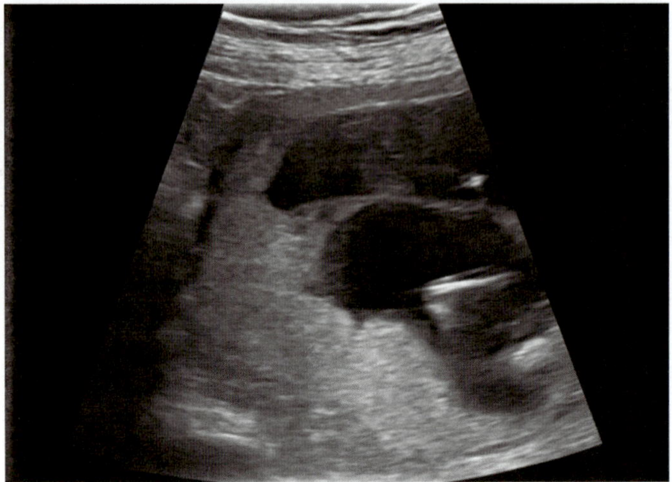

Fig. 3: Lambda sign—Dichorionicity.

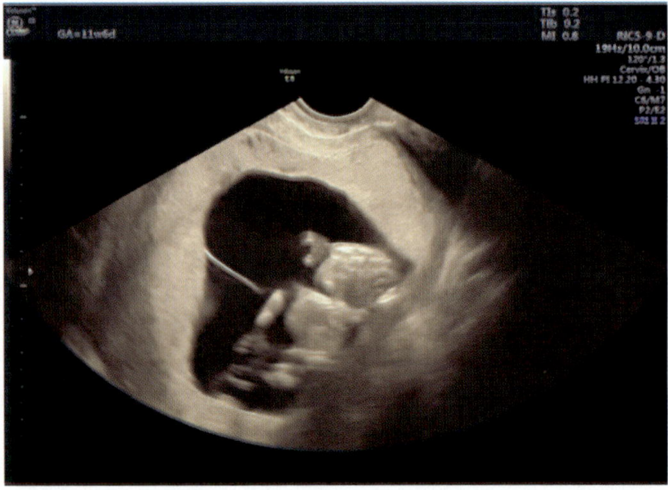

Fig. 4: T sign—Monochorionicity.

The placenta in midtrimester is evaluated for its general appearance, site with relationship to lower segment/internal os. While the site can be well established by transabdominal ultrasound in cases where the lower edge is seen clearly but in doubtful scenarios it is necessary to establish the distance of the lower edge of the placenta from the internal os by TVS. It is irresponsible to report low lying placenta without clearly demonstrating the lower edge in the lower segment and its distance from the cervical os by TVS in mid trimester ultrasound. **Figure 6** shows a complete placenta previa covering the internal os clearly seen by TVS.

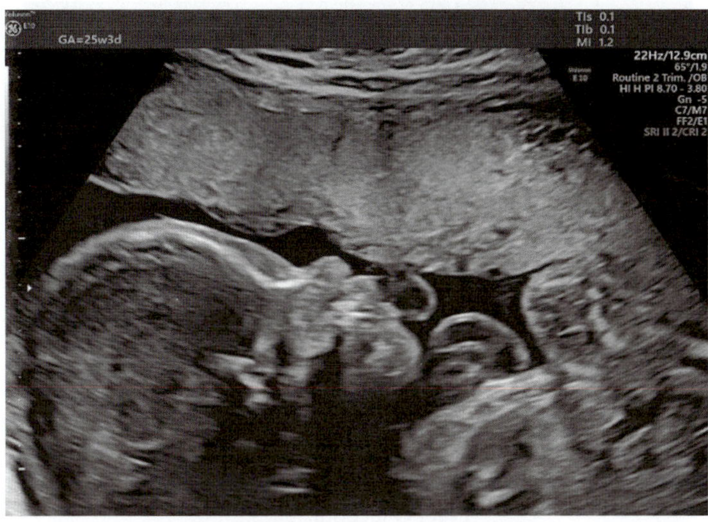

Fig. 5: Normal midtrimester placenta.

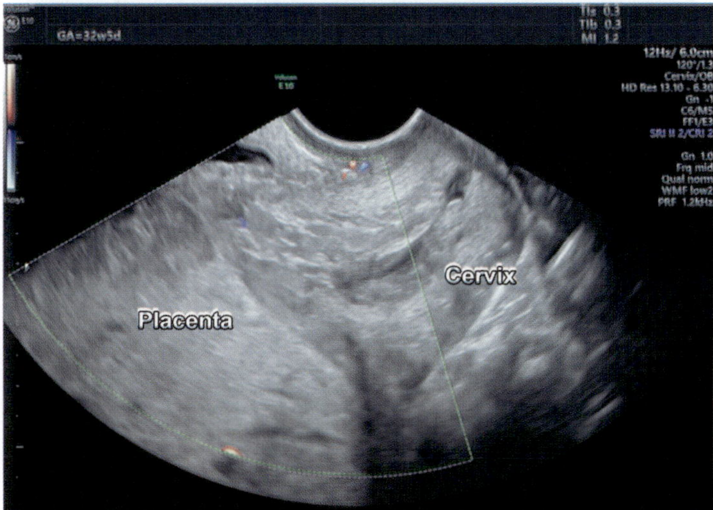

Fig. 6: Complete placenta previa.

Sometimes the placenta may ne normally positioned but may have structural abnormalities like lakes **(Fig. 7)**, mesenchymal dysplastic changes **(Fig. 8)** or tumors like chorangiomas **(Fig. 9)**

Abnormalities of the placenta in midtrimester will alert towards pregnancy complications. Placental lakes may be considered physiological if they constitute less than 10% of the entire placental mass but if they are significant, they are considered to be risk factors for placental dysfunction.

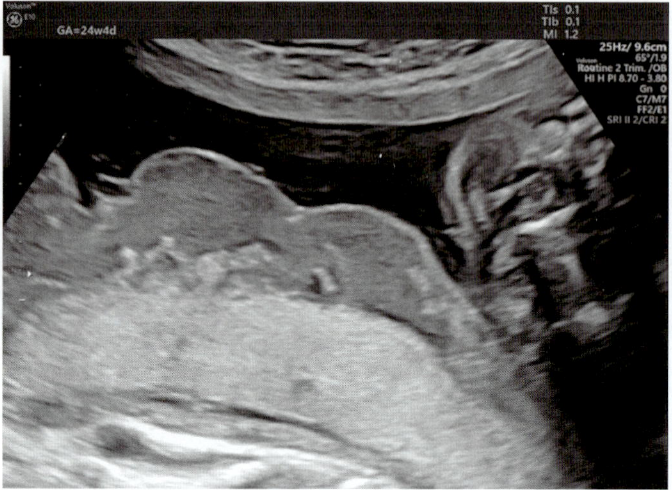

Fig. 7: Placental lakes.

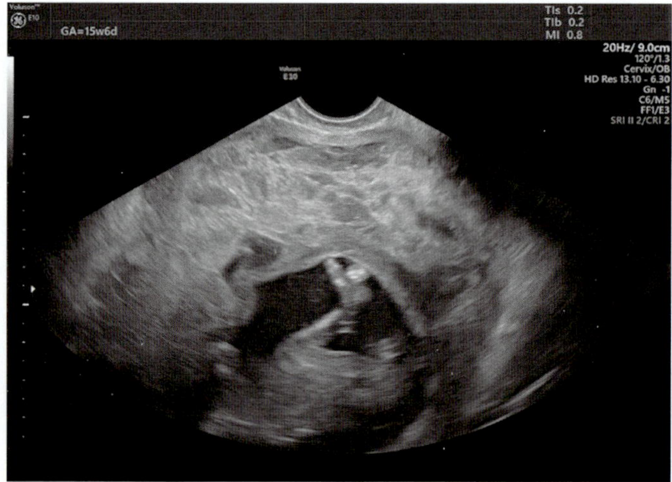

Fig. 8: Suggestive of mesenchymal dysplasia.

The variegated appearance of the placenta suggestive of mesenchymal dysplasia is rather commonly associated with severe early onset IUGR and poor perinatal outcomes.

Placental chorangiomas are tumors which may remain asymptomatic is small and non-progressive. However, if the chorangioma is progressively increasing in size or has a large feeding vessel then it can lead to polyhydramnios and fetal hydrops secondary to anemia due to sequestration of fetal erythrocytes in the tumor mass.

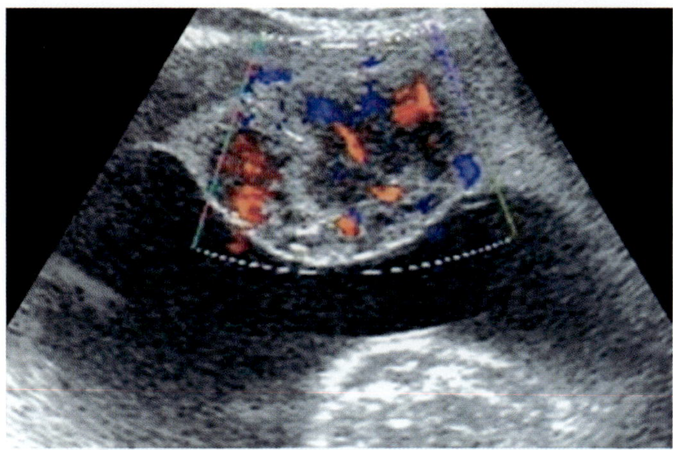

Fig. 9: Chorangioma.

In the present-day clinical scenario, ultrasound has made it possible to diagnose these placental abnormalities and help in prognostication and management also.

ASSESSMENT OF PLACENTAL ADHERENCE IN ADVANCED PREGNANCY

Appearance of the placenta and its location with relationship to the lower segment has been discussed in regard to establishing the possibility of placenta previa which is an important risk factor for perinatal complications. In the present-day obstetrics, an emerging placental complication sis that of morbid adherence of the placenta to the uterine wall and sometimes to adjoining pelvic structures too – the Placenta Accreta Spectrum disorders.[2]

The lack of a well-defined hypoechoic retroplacental layer is a sign of possibility of placenta accreta and hence the ultrasonologists must train their eyes to look for this retroplacental zone carefully during obstetric ultrasonography.

Ultrasonographic signs of morbidly adherent placentae include loss of retroplacental clear margins, presence of lacunae in the placental mass as shown in **Figure 10**. Loss of retroplacental clear zone, interruption in the vesicouterine interface, placental bulge in the bladder or focal exophytic masses strongly suggest morbid adherence of placenta on grey scale 2D ultrasound imaging.

The suspicion of placental adherence can be further clarified by enhancing the sensitivity of ultrasound using color Doppler techniques as shown in **Figure 11**. Enhanced uterovesical vascularity with bridging vessels or feeder vessel in lacuna are the color Doppler signs of PAS.[3]

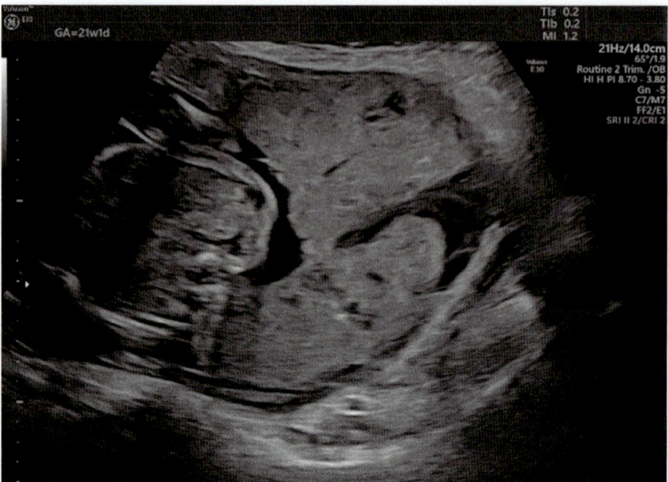

Fig. 10: Loss of retroplacental clear zone and presence of lacuna.

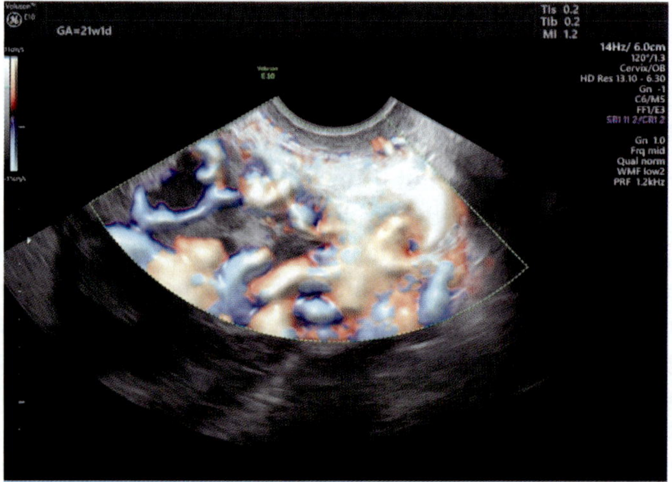

Fig. 11: Color Doppler enhancement to demonstrate PAS.

The modern ultrasound techniques allow for multiplanar display using combinations of 3D ultrasound and color Doppler to not only diagnose PAS but also clearly define the extent of adherence or invasion into adjoining tissues as shown in **Figure 12**.

The role of ultrasound in evaluation of Placenta Accreta Spectrum disorders has, revolutionized not only the diagnosis but also the management of the same. The FIGO grading system for PAS has been well established but its utility is only relevant from a surgical standpoint in **Table 1**. Today, ultrasound-based staging of PAS disorders is feasible and correlates

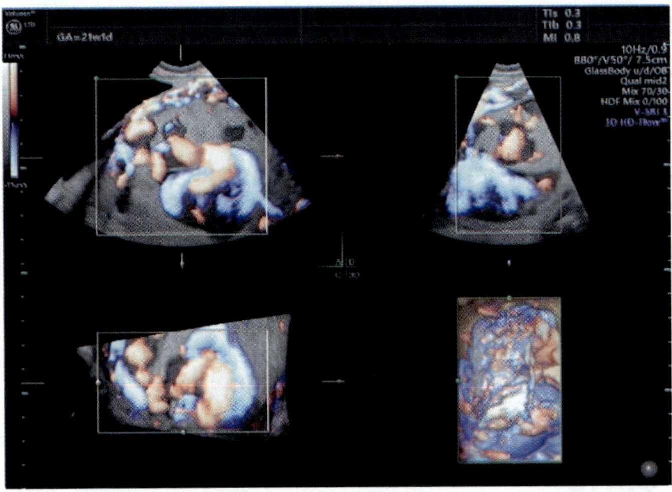

Fig. 12: 3D color Doppler enhancement for PAS.

TABLE 1: Representation for prenatal ultrasound-based staging of PAS disorders.

US stage of PAS disorder	*Ultrasound finding*	*Histopathology*	*FIGO grade*
PAS 0	• Placenta previa with no ultrasound signs of invasion or • Placenta previa with placental lacunae but no evidence of abnormal uterus-bladder interface (loss of clear zone and/or bladder wall interruption)	Placenta previa without PAS	1–2
PAS 1	Presence of at least two ultrasound signs among: • Placental lacunae • Loss of clear zone • Bladder wall interruption	Placental accrete/ increta	3
PAS 2	PAS1 plus uterovesical hypervascularity	Placenta percreta focal or diffuse	4–5
PAS 3	PAS1 or PAS2 plus evidence of increased vascularity in inferior part of lower uterine segment extending into parametrial region	Placenta percreta invading inferior third of lower uterine segment and lateral pelvic walls (or parametria)	6

with surgical outcome, depth of invasion and the FIGO clinical grading system.[4]

This staging system helps in planning intranatal care safely and helps in improving the overall perinatal outcomes.

CONCLUSION

- Placental evaluation MUST be part of every obstetric ultrasound as from early pregnancy till the time of delivery there are implications related to perinatal outcomes that can be directly attributed to the placenta.
- The position of the placenta must be clearly stated in the second trimester ultrasound and whenever there is suspicion of low lying placenta, TVS should be used to clearly define the diagnosis.
- Incidence of PAS is increasing in recent years and identifying ultrasound markers for PAS and high index of suspicion in high risk groups can help achieve reasonable prenatal diagnosis of PAS.
- Ultrasound staging system of PAS helps in planning definitive management and has been correlated with surgical outcomes.

KEY POINTS

- Ultrasound assessment of placental structure has gained importance in evaluation of pregnancy conditions that have implications on overall perinatal outcome.
- Starting from early pregnancy there are well defined parameters for structural assessment of placenta.
- In conditions like suspected adherence of placenta now ultrasound assessment can help diagnose the adherence with certainty and also help in establishing the degree of accreta hence helping in prognostication and planning surgery appropriately.
- Use of adjuncts like color Doppler technology greatly enhances the diagnostic potential of ultrasound in placental abnormalities.

REFERENCES

1. Schiffer V, van Haren A, De Cubber L, Bons J, Coumans A, van Kuijk SM, et al. Ultrasound evaluation of the placenta in healthy and placental syndrome pregnancies: A systematic review. Eur J Obstet Gynecol Reprod Biol. 2021;262: 45-56. doi: 10.1016/j.ejogrb.2021.04.042. Epub 2021 May 4. PMID: 33984727.
2. Jauniaux E, Collins S, Burton GJ. Placenta accreta spectrum: pathophysiology and evidence-based anatomy for prenatal ultrasound imaging. Am J Obstet Gynecol. 2018;218(1):75-87. doi: 10.1016/j.ajog.2017.05.067. Epub 2017 Jun 24. PMID: 28599899.
3. Horgan R, Abuhamad A. Placenta Accreta Spectrum: Prenatal Diagnosis and Management. Obstet Gynecol Clin North Am. 2022;49(3):423-38. doi: 10.1016/j.ogc.2022.02.004. PMID: 36122977.
4. Shainker SA, Coleman B, Timor-Tritsch IE, Bhide A, Bromley B, Cahill AG, et al. Society for Maternal-Fetal Medicine. Electronic address: pubs@smfm.org. Special Report of the Society for Maternal-Fetal Medicine Placenta Accreta Spectrum Ultrasound Marker Task Force: Consensus on definition of markers and approach to the ultrasound examination in pregnancies at risk for placenta accreta spectrum. Am J Obstet Gynecol. 2021;224(1):B2-B14. doi: 10.1016/j.ajog.2020.09.001. Erratum in: Am J Obstet Gynecol. 2021;225(1):91. doi: 10.1016/j.ajog.2021.02.012. PMID: 33386103.

CHAPTER

What is Better for Diagnosis: USG, CT or MRI?

Pratik Tambe, Deepti Gupta

INTRODUCTION

The female pelvic organs include the reproductive organs like the uterus, ovaries, and fallopian tubes, as well as the bladder and rectum. Gynecological pathologies encompass a diverse spectrum of conditions affecting female reproductive system, ranging from benign conditions like uterine fibroids/ endometriosis to life threatening malignancies like cervical and ovarian cancers.

The standardized Disability adjusted life years (DALYs) score for combined gynecological diseases (CGDs) ranged from 0.28 to 0.53% among women of childbearing age between 1990 to 2021[1]. DALYs and death of malignant gynecological tumors are most significant in women aged 40–49 years. Hence, it is imperative that screening and diagnosis of various common pelvic pathologies should be robust to expedite early diagnosis and treatment. This chapter aims to critically assess and compare the various imaging modalities in common pelvic pathologies and few common gynecological malignancies.

Modern radiology offers multiple modalities: Ultrasound (US) remains the frontline tool, computed tomography (CT) and magnetic resonance imaging (MRI) provide additional information, while 3D ultrasound adds volumetric precision. This comprehensive analysis synthesizes current evidence to compare these technologies for specific pelvic pathologies, incorporating diagnostic accuracy, clinical utility, and evolving guidelines.

FIBROID UTERUS

The most common benign tumor of female reproductive system are Uterine fibroids or leiomyomas. They are present in 20–30% women of reproductive age group.[2] Presenting symptoms vary include heavy menstrual flow, abnormal uterine bleeding, pelvic pain, adverse pregnancy outcomes and subfertility in some.

Adverse perinatal outcomes are often associated with fibroids, including preterm labor, low birth weight, placenta previa, placental abruption, obstructed labor, intrauterine growth restriction, caesarean section, postpartum hemorrhage, and postpartum maternal anemia. The diagnosis is largely based on history and clinical examination, but imaging modalities play crucial role in confirming the diagnosis, ruling out other differential diagnoses and take recourse to myoma mapping to aid the future treatment plan.

Role of Ultrasound (USG)

Ultrasound is the first line investigation for uterine fibroid and USG features suggestive of fibroid include well-defined, spherical, solid, heterogenous lesion within the myometrium, relatively hypoechoic from neighboring myometrium, often the edges of the lesion show acoustic shadowing. A circumferential flow around the lesion is often visible on color Doppler. Ideally examination should include both transvaginal ultrasound (TVUS) and transabdominal scan.

Figure 1 demonstrates a fibroid on transvaginal 2 D ultrasound while **Figure 2** shows the peripheral vascularity on color Doppler imaging in same lesion.

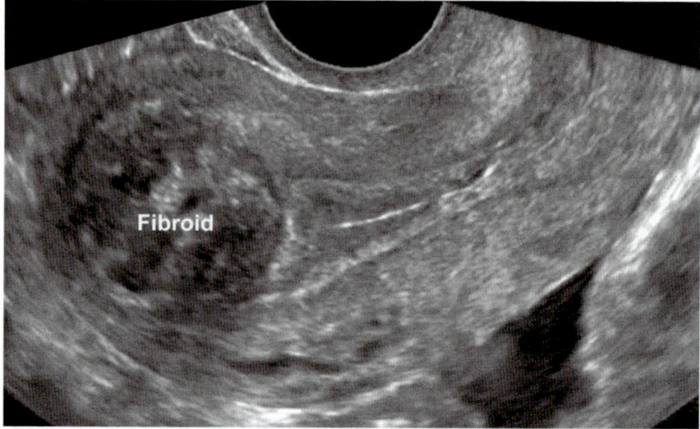

Fig. 1: Fundal fibroid on 2D transvaginal ultrasound.

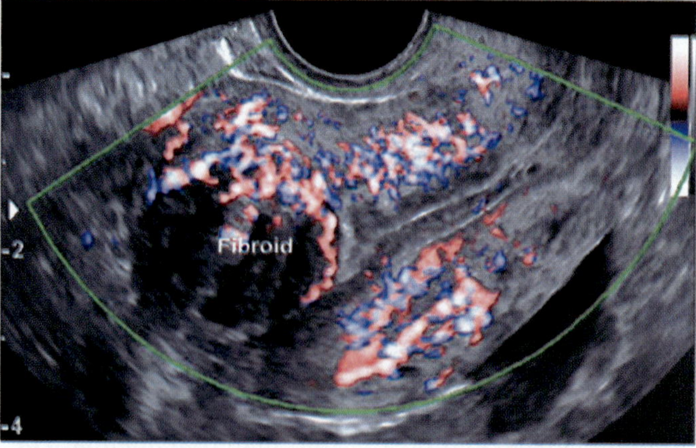

Fig. 2: Peripheral vascularity of same fibroid on color Doppler.

Differential Diagnosis

Adenomyosis especially focal may sometimes be confused with an intramural myoma. Few Features which suggest presence of adenomyosis include enlarged globular uterus, absence of leiomyomata, anechoic cystic spaces or lakes in the myometrium, echoic linear striations in sub-endometrial location, thickened uterine wall, heterogeneous echo texture, blurring of endometrial-myometrial junction and thickening of the transition zone.[3]

Subserous fibroids can be confused with ovarian masses especially the solid/fibrous variety like Brenner tumor and fibrothecoma. A circumferential vascularity, blood flow, and arterial supply on color Doppler helps in establishing diagnosis of fibroid. Similarly submucous myoma can be confused with endometrial polyps. Multiple, circular feeding vessels are characteristic for fibroids, whereas a single feeding artery can be observed in most polyps. Ideally, both transvaginal and transabdominal ultrasound must be performed for good mapping and ruling out subserosal/other adnexal masses.

Role of Computed Tomography (CT) Scan

CT-Scan is not a preferred modality for uterine fibroids and diagnosis of fibroid is often incidental. Fibroids show low attenuation relative to the myometrium on contrast-enhanced scans.

Role of Magnetic Resonance Imaging (MRI)

MRI is preferred investigation for accurately identifying pelvic pathologies. When ordered for uterine fibroids, MRI sequences should include both sagittal and axial sequences in T1 weighted (T1W) and T2 weighted (T2W) images.

Expected findings on MRI include[4] a high signal intensity for normal endometrium, low signal band showing junctional zone and inner myometrium, intermediate signals of remainder myometrium. The fibroids are seen as low-signal intensity, well defined masses as compared to the myometrium on T2W images and isointense to the myometrium on T1W images. There may also be a high-intensity rim which is seen on T2W images.

Figure 3 shows an MRI T2W image depicting a large fibroid.

DEGENERATING MYOMAS

Findings suggestive of various degenerative changes are different in different types of degenerations. Hyaline degeneration appears as low signal on T2W images, with no enhancement. On other hand, cystic degeneration appears as high-signal intensity on T2W images and low-signal on T1W images. Contrary to both, recent hemorrhagic degeneration can be seen as high signal on both T1W and T2W images.

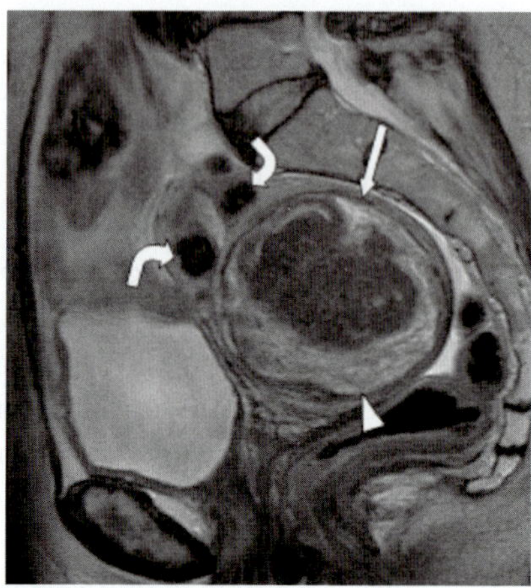

Fig. 3: MRI T2W image with arrow pointing to low intensity fibroid and arrowhead pointing to high intensity rim.

USG versus MRI for Myomas

MRI has a special role in uterine fibroids as it is more sensitive, there is no use of ionizing radiation. It demonstrates zonal anatomy with detection of small fibroids, and identification of fibroids in relatively unusual locations is possible.

According to Levens et al., positive predictive value (PPV) of MRI was 91% (95% CI: 85%, 95%). The sensitivity was 80% (95% CI: 73%, 86%) for detection of fibroids. On other hand, PPV for ultrasound was 97% (95% CI: 89%, 100%) and sensitivity for US was 40% (95% CI: 32%, 48%), respectively[5].

Another study concluded that both MRI and 3D USG were 100% accurate in women with <5 fibroids. However, MRI was more accurate in the detection and removal of all fibroids in patients with >4 fibroids (sensitivity 94% vs. 87%, $p < 0.05$) which also correlated with a larger uterus.[6]

CERVICAL CANCER

Cervical cancer primarily affects women of reproductive age group. Even though staging of cervical cancer is clinical, there is wide use of imaging techniques like CT, MRI, positron emission tomography-CT (PET-CT). Additional imaging is often used for assessing important prognostic factors like size of tumor, parametrial involvement, endocervical extension, involvement of pelvic side wall or adjacent/distal organs and lymph node status. Apart from these, few clinical situations where additional imaging may be needed are follow-up of cervical cancer, evaluating tumor response to treatment, and selection of suitable patients with early stage disease who may be fit for less radical surgeries like radical trachelectomy for fertility preservation.

Ultrasound

Ultrasound has limited role in cervical cancer management and follow-up.

CT-Scan

CT accuracy is reported to range from 32-80% for overall cervical cancer staging. It is not reliable for assessing local spread because of PPV for detection of early parametrial invasion being lower than 58%.[7] As of now, patients with clinical evidence of advanced disease or contraindications to MRI may be offered staging with CT.

Magnetic Resonance Imaging

On MRI imaging, normal cervical stroma is hypointense. On T2 weighted images, in contrast Cervical cancer appears as a moderately hyperintense area. T2W sequences demonstrate tumor extension to the parametrial fat in a better way. Parametrial involvement can be excluded with a finding of >3 mm T2 hypointense stromal cervical rim, as it has extremely high specificity (96–99%) and NPV (94–100%)[7].

CT versus MRI for Cervical Cancer

MRI is the preferred imaging modality for following reasons. The rationale for the same relies on contrast resolution is high, differentiation between cancerous and normal tissues is more accurate with accuracy values 75–96% and it has high negative predictive value (94–100%) for involvement of parametria.

MRI is safe and when it comes to assessing tumor extension to uterine corpus, it has high sensitivity (86–91%) and specificity (94–96%). There is moderate sensitivity and specificity for both CT and MRI (43–73%) as regards detection of metastatic lymph nodes because of inability to distinguish between inflammatory enlarged and metastatic lymph nodes.

Special Situations

In postoperative women, no imaging recommended in surgically treated early-stage disease. A combination of MRI and PET-CT is preferred for the diagnosis of cervical cancer relapse. MRI should be performed at least ten days after a biopsy, to avoid false positive results due to local inflammation.

OVARIAN CANCER

Indian Council of Medical Research (ICMR) estimates an age-adjusted incidence rate of ovarian cancer of around 6.8 per 100,000 women.[8]

In ovarian neoplasm, pre-operative imaging aims to:

- Help predict benign, borderline, or malignant subtypes

- Differentiate organ of origin as ovary or the adnexa
- Evaluate for metastatic disease.

Ultrasound

The first line imaging modality in confirmed/suspected adnexal mass is ultrasound. It should ideally be transvaginal and transabdominal scan. Ovarian-Adnexal Reporting and Data System (O-RADS), US risk stratification and International Ovarian Tumour Analysis (IOTA) are used for risk stratification using ultrasound features. **Table 1** depicts the O-RADS vs. IOTA classification systems.

CT-Scan

CT remains the recommended modality for staging of ovarian cancer. Primary applications of CT in ovarian neoplasm are the preoperative staging and restaging after debulking surgery for malignant neoplasms. Apart from these, CT may be used when complications from ovarian cancer are suspected. The key roles for CT-Scan include staging of ovarian cancer, operability, identification of lesions in areas that are difficult to resect. It also characterizes the tubo-ovarian lesion, detects the involvement of the adjacent pelvic organs and also detects the extension of the disease outside the pelvis. In patients undergoing neoadjuvant chemotherapy prior to interval debulking, it helps to assess response to treatment. It also helps to detect recurrence.

For detecting recurrence, CECT is reported to have sensitivity of 58–84% and specificity of 59–100%. In staging of ovarian cancer, reported accuracy of CT is up to 94%.[10]

Magnetic Resonance Imaging

MRI offers superior contrast resolution. When compared to USG/CT, MRI is a superior modality in the evaluation of indeterminate adnexal lesions. Compared to USG, MRI has increased specificity which decreases the number of false-positive diagnoses for malignancy and therefore avoids unnecessary or over-extensive surgery. The accuracy to CT in staging of ovarian cancer is considered equivalent to MRI, with sensitivity of 0.88, specificity of 0.74, and accuracy of 0.84. However, MRI has certain limitations as it is more sensitive to motion and has long duration of study compared to CT.[10]

ENDOMETRIAL CANCER

With an incidence of about 4.3 per 100,000 women, endometrial cancer is the second most common gynecological malignancy in India and developing countries.[11] There are many known risk factors like Obesity, unopposed estrogen intake, nulliparity, diabetes mellitus, Stein–Leventhal

TABLE 1: O-RADS vs IOTA classification systems.[9]

O-RADS score	Risk category [IOTA model]	Lexicon descriptors		Premenopausal management	Postmenopausal management
0	Incomplete evaluation (N/A)	N/A		Repeat study or alternate study	
1	Normal Ovary (N/A)	Follicle defined as a simple cyst ≤ 3 cm Corpus luteum ≤ 3 cm		None	N/A
2	Almost certainly benign (<1%)	Simple cyst	≤ 3 cm > 3–5 cm > 5 but <10 cm	N/A None Follow-up in 8–12 weeks	None Follow up in 1 year *
		Classic Benign Lesions	For separate descriptors		
		Non-simple unilocular cyst, smooth inner margin	≤ 3 cm > 3 but < 10 cm	None Follow-up in 8–12 weeks if concerning, US specialist or MRI	Follow up in 1 year* if concerning, US specialist or MRI US specialist or MRI
3	Low risk malignancy (1–<10%)	• Unilocular cyst ≥ 10 cm (simple or non-simple) • Typical dermoid cysts, endometriomas, hemorrhagic cysts ≥ 10 cm • Unilocular cyst, any size with irregular inner wall < 3 mm height • Multilocular cyst < 10 cm, smooth inner wall, CS = 1–3 • Solid smooth, any size, CS = 1			US specialist or MRI Management by gynecologist
4	Immediate risk (10–<50%)	Multilocular cyst, no solid component	≥ 10 cm, smooth inner wall, CS = 1–3 Any size, smooth inner wall, CS = 4 Any size, irregular inner wall and/or irregular septation, any color score		US specialist or MRI
		Unilocular cyst with solid component	Any size, 0–3 papillary projections		Management by gynecologist with GYN-oncologist consultation or solely by GYN-oncologist
		Multilocular cyst with solid component	Any size. CS = 1–2		
		Solid	Smooth, any size, CS = 2-3		
5	High risk (≥ 50%)	Unilocular cyst, any size. CS = any Multilocular cyst with solid component, any size, CS = 3–4 Solid smooth, any size, CS = 4 Ascites and/or peritoneal nodules			GYN-oncologist

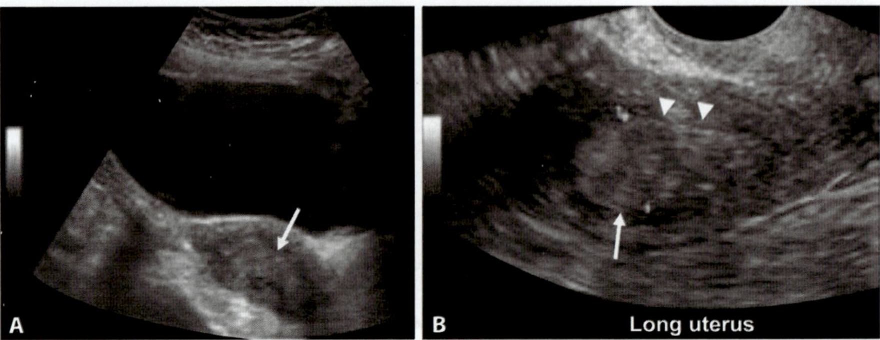

Figs. 4A and B: TVUS appearance showing thickened endometrium in EC with arrowheads showing intact endomyometrial junction.

syndrome, Lynch syndrome, and tamoxifen therapy. An endometrial biopsy aids definitive diagnosis. Histologically it is of two types-endometrioid adenocarcinoma (type I) that accounts for 90% of the tumors and Type II ECs include the clear-cell, serous papillary subtypes and carcinosarcomas.

Ultrasound

In symptomatic women, initial evaluation is done by transvaginal ultrasound because it is inexpensive, easily available and devoid of ionizing radiation. For detecting EC, TVUS has sensitivity and specificity of 96% and 61%, respectively. An endometrial thickness threshold of 5 mm is used in the postmenopausal women. A meta-analysis suggested a sensitivity of 68-100% and a specificity of 71-90% for subjective assessment of deep myometrial invasion.[12]

TVUS has reported sensitivity and specificity of 69% and 70%, respectively in determining the depth of myometrial invasion. Color Doppler when used reveals increased vascularity but has limited role in differentiating from benign pathologies.

Figures 4A and B TVUS appearance in case of endometrial cancer in a woman with postmenopausal bleeding.

CT-Scan

EC appears as hypoattenuating and hypo enhancing mass in the endometrial cavity on a contrast enhanced CT-Scan. Submucosal leiomyomas, endometrial polyps, or cervical stenosis maybe differential diagnosis with similar picture. Compared to MRI, CT-Scan is less sensitive and less specific in accurate visualization of myometrial invasion and cervical involvement. The sensitivity and specificity of CT in evaluating myometrial invasion is 40–83% and from 42–75%, respectively.[10]

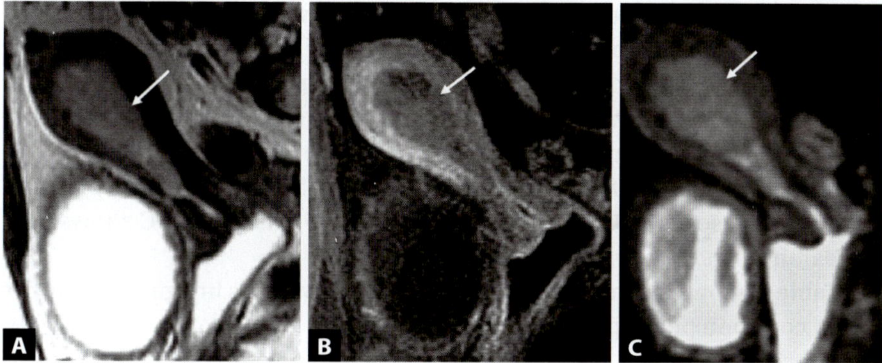

Figs. 5A to C: MRI in a case of EC- hyperintense signal on T2W and isointense on T1W sequence.

TABLE 2: Imaging modalities in gynecological conditions.

Pathology	*USG*	*CT-Scan*	*MRI*
Uterine fibroids	1st investigation	Limited utility	Recommended in cases with large fibroid volume/>5 myomas/ difficult locations/ young patient desirous of uterus preserving surgery
Cervical cancer	Diagnosis and staging-clinical	Limited role	Preferred to assess local extent of disease
Ovarian cancer	1st investigation, O-RADS/IOTA tools used for risk stratification	Preferred modality for disease staging	Recommended in indeterminate adnexal mass
Endometrial cancer	1st investigation	Limited utility	Recommended for disease staging and myometrial invasion assessment

Magnetic Resonance Imaging

MRI is the most accurate imaging modality for the local staging of EC prior to treatment, owing to its excellent soft tissue delineation is MRI. On T1 weighted images, hypo-to-isointense mass is suggestive of EC whereas on T2 weighted images, intermediate signal intensity lower than the normal endometrium is suggestive of EC. The overall staging accuracy of MR imaging is reported to be 83-92%.

T2W sequences give optimal depiction of myometrial invasion. The accuracy can be further enhanced by using dynamic contrast enhanced MRI

(DCE-MRI). The negative predictive value of dynamic contrast enhanced MRI is better than the positive predictive value for myometrial invasion.

Thinning of the myometrium in postmenopausal women, tumor extension into the cornua, myometrial compression from a polypoid tumor and presence of leiomyomas or adenomyosis maybe limiting factors in the MRI evaluation of EC. The sensitivity of MRI for picking up lymph node metastases is 44% and specificity is 98%. **Figures 5A to C** shows MRI appearances in EC.

Table 2 shows a comparison and the utility of various imaging modalities in few common pelvic pathologies.

CONCLUSION

There is a wide range of imaging modalities available in diagnostic armamentarium. It is prudent to make judicious use in order to extract maximum information in least cost and time to aid patient management. While ultrasound remains the first choice in uterine myomas, in cervical cancer MRI may be utilized to assess degree and extent of spread.

CT finds extensive application in evaluation of ovarian tumors and cancers, as an adjunct to ultrasound. MRI is the preferred modality for endometrial cancers with an aim for assessment of myometrial invasion and disease spread, in addition to transvaginal ultrasound.

Newer modalities like PET-CT continue to aid our understanding of these conditions and where appropriate, available and affordable, may be incorporated into the management workflow to enhance patient outcomes and survival.

KEY POINTS

- There are various imaging modalities for evaluation of Gynecological pathologies like ultrasound, CT scan, MRI.
- Ultrasound is first investigation of choice in fibroids, supplemented with MRI in special situations.
- In cases of carcinoma cervix, ultrasound has limited role and MRI is preferred imaging technique.
- For evaluation of ovarian/adnexal masses, ultrasound with CECT is preferred.
- Endometrial carcinoma is best evaluated by TVUS followed by MRI.
- TVS should always be combined with abdominal scan as well for thorough and complete assessment of pelvic Gynecological pathology.

REFERENCES

1. Gao Y, Wang X, Wang Q, Jiang L, Wu C, Guo Y, et al. Rising global burden of common gynecological diseases in women of childbearing age from 1990 to

2021: an update from the Global Burden of Disease Study 2021. Reprod Health. 2025;22(1):57. doi: 10.1186/s12978-025-02013-1. PMID: 40259342; PMCID: PMC12010537.

2. Sabry M, Al-Hendy A. Medical treatment of uterine leiomyoma. Reproductive sciences (Thousand Oaks, Calif). 2012;19:339-53.
3. Sakhel K, Abuhamad A. Sonography of adenomyosis. J Ultrasound Med. 2012;31:805-8. doi: 10.7863/jum.2012.31.5.805. [DOI] [PubMed]
4. Wilde S, Scott-Barrett S. Radiological appearances of uterine fibroids. Indian J Radiol Imaging. 2009;19(3):222-31. doi: 10.4103/0971-3026.54887. PMID: 19881092; PMCID: PMC2766886.
5. Levens ED, Wesley R, Premkumar A, Blocker W, Nieman LK. Magnetic resonance imaging and transvaginal ultrasound for determining fibroid burden: implications for research and clinical care. Am J Obstet Gynecol. 2009;200(5):537.e1-7. doi: 10.1016/j.ajog.2008.12.037. Epub 2009 Mar 9. PMID: 19268886; PMCID: PMC2701348.
6. Stadtmauer L. The accuracy of 3D ultrasound and MRI in predicting the number of fibroids removed with robot assisted laparoscopic myomectomy. Fertility and Sterility, Volume 108, Issue 3, e261-e262.
7. Bourgioti C, Chatoupis K, Moulopoulos LA. Current imaging strategies for the evaluation of uterine cervical cancer. World J Radiol. 2016;8(4):342-54. doi: 10.4329/wjr.v8.i4.342. PMID: 27158421; PMCID: PMC4840192.
8. Rajendra Kumar Meena et al. Patterns of treatment and outcomes in epithelial ovarian cancer: a retrospective North Indian Single-Institution Experience. JCO Glob Oncol. 2022;8:e2200032. DOI:10.1200/GO.22.00032.
9. Andreotti RF, Timmerman D, Strachowski LM, Froyman W, Benacerraf BR, Bennett GL, et al. O-RADS US Risk Stratification and Management System: A Consensus Guideline from the ACR Ovarian-Adnexal Reporting and Data System Committee. Radiology. 2020;294(1):168-85. doi: 10.1148/radiol.2019191150. Epub 2019 Nov 5. PMID: 31687921.
10. Renganathan R, Prema R, Popat P, Manchanda S, Venkatesh KA, Chandramohan A, et al. Imaging recommendations for diagnosis, staging, and management of ovarian and fallopian tube cancers. Indian J Med Paediatr Oncol. 2023;44. 10.1055/s-0042-1759518.
11. Faria SC, Sagebiel T, Balachandran A, Devine C, Lal C, Bhosale PR. Imaging in endometrial carcinoma. Indian J Radiol Imaging. 2015;25(2):137-47. doi: 10.4103/0971-3026.155857. PMID: 25969637; PMCID: PMC4419423.
12. Epstein E, Blomqvist L. Imaging in endometrial cancer. Best Pract Res Clin Obstet Gynaecol. 2014;28:721–39. doi: 10.1016/j.bpobgyn.2014.04.007.

CHAPTER

Role of Artificial Intelligence in Imaging

Archana Baser, Anshu Baser

INTRODUCTION

Artificial imaging (AI) is increasingly being adapted into medical practice worldwide. There are now many hospitals that are using AI from diagnosis to treatment starting from Hospital Management Systems to diagnosis and treatment.

In the context of Imaging there is increasing data suggesting that AI has excellent accuracy in detecting small radiographic abnormalities.[1]

Let us now look individually into the various imaging modalities in the medical field and see the role of AI.

ULTRASONOGRAPHY

Ultrasound is one of the most widely used investigations especially in the field of gynecology.

AI has been used in various aspects of ultrasonography. It has been used for thyroid, musculoskeletal and breast tissue. AI has application in enhancing quality of ultrasound images, images, automated report generations based on ultrasonographic images; determining quantitative or predictive data from images, which is difficult for a human operator to do based on visual observations; and dividing the ultrasound images automatically into sections to improve efficiency. This list of AI applications to ultrasonography is expected to increase the future.[2]

AI is particularly useful for less experienced examiners and can improve diagnostic accuracy.[3]

Ultrasound is more used modality than magnetic resonance imaging (MRI) and computed tomography (CT) and is typically an operator dependent investigation.

This in turn increases variability between examiners and subjectivity of ultrasound compared to CT MRI.

In this regard, AI offers a unique opportunity to improve performance of ultrasonography by removing interobserver variability. However because ultrasound is an operator dependent modality developing AI for the same is challenging. There are a few problems with AI in ultrasonography. Ultrasound is real time so therefore it requires a highly sophisticated AI system and an experienced operator to provide adequate image input for AI systems to generate an output.

The final images rendered in the report are also dependent on the operator and hence increase variability and limit application of AI.[4]

COMPUTED TOMOGRAPHY

There has been a rapid evolution in computed tomography (CT) has lead to increasing no of CT scans being performed regularly. CT scans improve diagnostic efficacy, reduce uncertainty and facilitate timely intervention.

However CT scans have the potential disadvantage of higher radiation exposure and there is rising concern regarding radiation induced cancer.[5]

In an effort to reduce this various methods have been investigated image reconstruction is one of those techniques. Artificial intelligence is an upcoming modality in CT image reconstruction that is being developed with the goal of further dose reduction through improved image quality. Some examples of AI application in radiology include detection of polyps in colonoscopy, identification of pulmonary nodules in lung cancer, and assistance with interpretation of mammography images for micro-calcifications.[6]

MAGNETIC RESONANCE IMAGING[7]

1. Enhanced image acquisition and processing:
    - *Accelerated imaging:* AI algorithms can reconstruct images from less data, significantly speeding up MRI scans without compromising image quality.
    - *Automated patient positioning:* AI can identify anatomical landmarks and guide the patient's position within the scanner, reducing setup time and improving consistency.
    - *Improved image quality:* AI can enhance image quality by correcting artifacts, optimizing protocols, and using adaptive sampling techniques.
    - *Faster scan times:* AI-powered algorithms can reduce scan times by up to 50% while maintaining image quality, allowing for more patients to be scanned in the same timeframe.
2. AI-driven image analysis:
    - *Tumor detection and characterization:* AI can identify and characterize tumors in MRI scans, aiding in early detection and staging.
    - *Neurological disorder diagnosis:* AI algorithms can assist in diagnosing neurological disorders like Alzheimer's by analyzing brain MRI scans.
    - *Cardiovascular assessment:* AI can be used to assess cardiac function, detect heart disease, and guide treatment decisions in cardiology.

- *Incidental finding detection:* AI can help identify incidental findings (like nodules) on MRI scans, preventing radiologists from overlooking important information.

3. Improved clinical decision-making:
    - *Assisted reporting:* AI can assist radiologists with reporting by identifying key findings and flagging suspicious areas, streamlining the reporting process.
    - *Predictive analytics:* AI can be used to predict patient wait times for MRI and other imaging modalities.
    - *Image-guided interventions:* AI can enhance surgical precision and reduce procedural risks by providing surgeons with real-time imaging and navigation assistance.

CONCLUSION

AI is now booming and it is now expected to develop into more accurate and less expensive versions in the medical field making it more and more accessible with each passing day.

The aim is not only to increase efficiency but to focus on patient centered care and precision.[8]

KEY POINTS

- AI helps reduce interobserver variability.
- There are now increasing applications of AI including AI assisted pre pick up screening.
- AI in ultrasound is still evolving due to dynamic nature of ultrasound.
- AI is inevitable let us embrace it rather than erase it.

REFERENCES

1. Oren O, Gersh BJ, Bhatt DL. Artificial intelligence in medical imaging: switching from radiographic pathological data to clinically meaningful endpoints. Lancet Digit Health. 2020;2(9):e486-e488. doi: 10.1016/S2589-7500(20)30160-6. PMID: 33328116
2. Park SH. Artificial intelligence for ultrasonography: unique opportunities and challenges. Ultrasonography. 2021;40(1):3-6. doi: 10.14366/usg.20078. Epub 2020 Nov 3. PMID: 33227844; PMCID: PMC7758099.
3. Jeong Y, Kim JH, Chae HD, Park SJ, Bae JS, Joo I, et al. Deep learning-based decision support system for the diagnosis of neoplastic gallbladder polyps on ultrasonography: preliminary results. Sci Rep. 2020;10:7700. doi: 10.1038/s41598-020-64205-y.
4. Park SH, Han K. Methodologic guide for evaluating clinical performance and effect of artificial intelligence technology for medical diagnosis and prediction. Radiology. 2018;286:800-9. doi: 10.1148/radiol.2017171920. [DOI] [PubMed] [Google Scholar]

5. Zhang Z, Seeram E. The use of artificial intelligence in computed tomography image reconstruction - A literature review. J Med Imaging Radiat Sci. 2020;51(4):671-677. doi: 10.1016/j.jmir.2020.09.001. Epub 2020 Sep 24.
6. Hosny A, Parmar C, Quackenbush J, Schwartz LH, Aerts HJWL. Artificial intelligence in radiology. Nat Rev Cancer. 2018;18(8):500-10. doi: 10.1038/s41568-018-0016-5. PMID: 29777175; PMCID: PMC6268174.
7. Shimron E, Perlman O. AI in MRI: Computational frameworks for a faster, optimized, and automated imaging workflow. Bioengineering (Basel). 2023;10(4):492. doi: 10.3390/bioengineering10040492. PMID: 37106679; PMCID: PMC10135995.
8. Malamateniou C, Knapp KM, Pergola M, Woznitza N, Hardy M. Artificial intelligence in radiography: Where are we now and what does the future hold?, Radiography (Lond). 2021;27 Suppl 1:S58-S62. ISSN 1078-8174, https://doi.org/10.1016/j.radi.2021.07.015.(https://www.sciencedirect.com/science/article/pii/S107881742100095X)

Index

Page numbers followed by *f* refer to figure and *t* refer to table.

N

O

P

Q

R